SLED

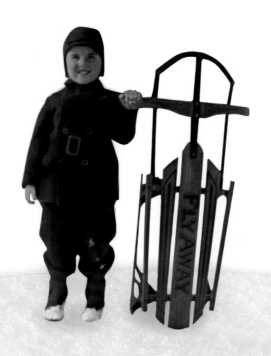

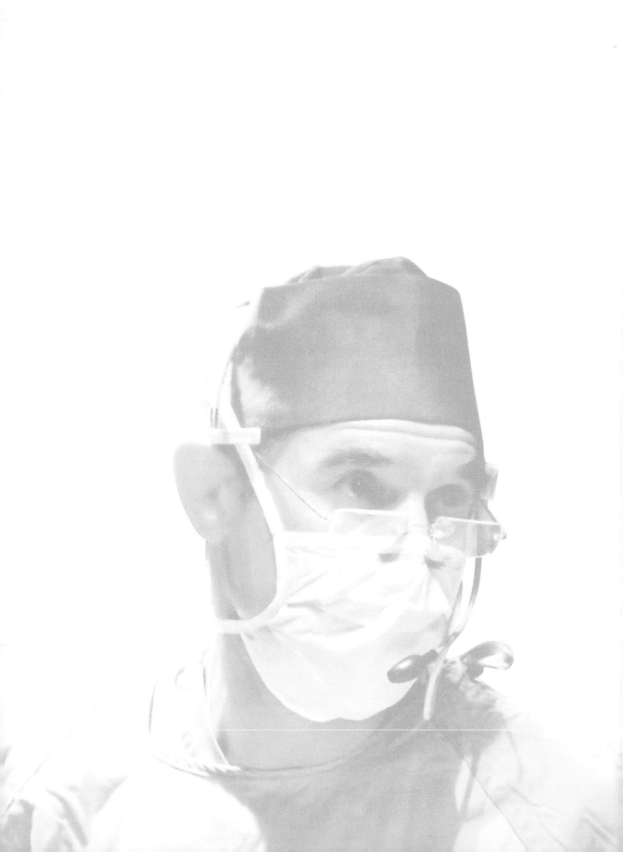

SLED

The
Serendipitous Life of Edward Diethrich

Edward B. Diethrich, MD

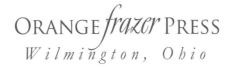

ORANGE *frazer* PRESS

Wilmington, Ohio

ISBN 978-1939710-406
Copyright©2016 Edward B. Diethrich
All Rights Reserved

Published for the author by:
Orange Frazer Press
P.O. Box 214
Wilmington, OH 45177

Telephone: 937.382.3196 for price and shipping information.
Website: www.orangefrazer.com or www.drteddiethrich.com

Book and cover design: Alyson Rua and Orange Frazer Press

*Photo on page 10 attributed to Otis Historical Archives National
Museum of Health and Medicine*

Library of Congress Control Number: 2015958573

Printed in the United States of America.

To all my friends, colleagues, and patients throughout the world who made this endeavor possible, my deepest appreciation.

And finally to my family, Gloria, Tad, and Lynne who tolerated me throughout this ride.

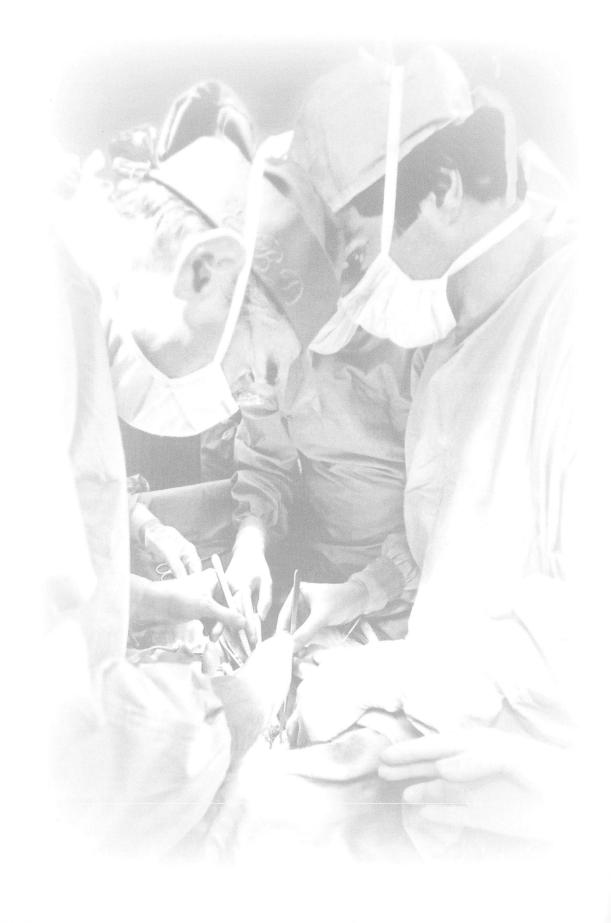

Acknowledgments

A special thanks to Paula Banahan, RN, for her extraordinary project management; Rebecca Bowman for her expert editorial advice; Lauren Wise for her early explorations and editorial comments; Nancy Ashland for manuscript assembly; Tony Forner for his unique talent in photographic artistry; and Kelli Kent for her ability to read my writing.

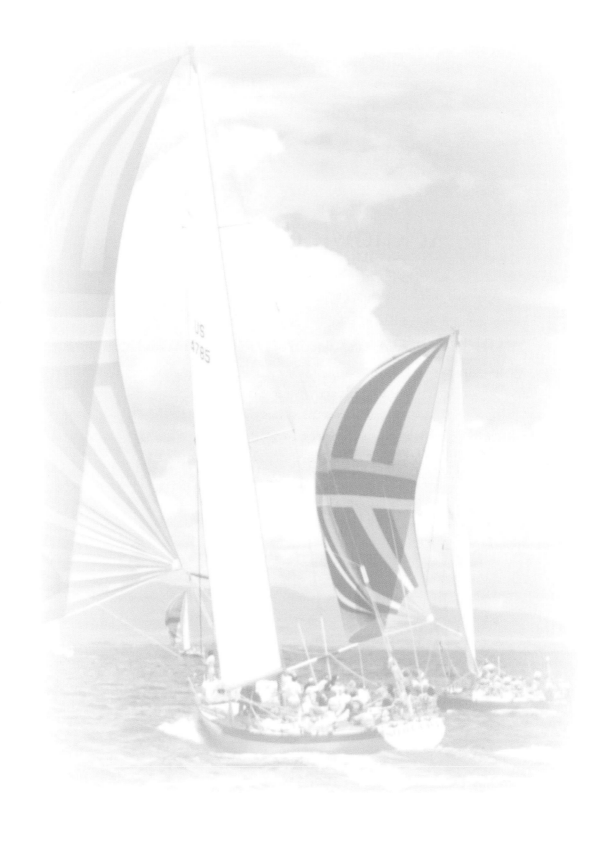

Contents

Preface

Among my friends and family, this manuscript has been titled, "The Serendipitous Life of Edward Diethrich" for quite some time. It embodies the fortuitousness of my life and the discoveries, both personal and reputable, along the way. Even the acronym S.L.E.D. has meaning to me, as you'll see in the Introduction.

Why use a term like "serendipitous" when illuminating the career of a heart surgeon? After all, as illustrated early on in this book, our training is highly structured, and our internships, residencies, and post-graduate training are pretty much "stamped" with board and society approval. Requirements such as these are very much in contrast to serendipity, where one makes desirable discoveries by accident or sagacity.

When my father provided me with a copy of the Louisa May Alcott cookbook, I wondered if maybe I was created with her aptitude gene. The cookbook came with a note explaining that Bronson Alcott, father of Louisa, was a first cousin of my

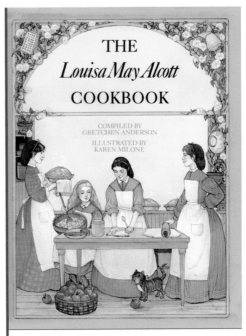

Louisa May Alcott Cookbook.

Dear Gloria—

A little bit of family trick from my Mother's side.

Bronson Alcott, the father of Louisa May was a first cousin of Ted's Great, Great Grandfather James Bronson, Sr.

Not such a much as a Cook Book, but maybe a Keepsake

Love
Dad.

This note was included in the cookbook sent to Gloria from my father.

great-great-grandfather James Bronson Sr., hence my middle name: Edward Bronson Diethrich.

Of interest is that Louisa May Alcott served as a nurse in the Civil War, carried a love for music her entire life, and fashioned herself a tomboy, choosing to enjoy outdoor activities better suited for boys. How fitting to learn that this world-renowned author also lived her life with the same three passions as I: medicine, music, and sports.

But as we have so recently learned, those genes can raise havoc with all of our lives. No life—and no person, for that matter—is meant to be perfect. It's the challenges along the way that really allow others to benefit from our story.

Early on in life I was afforded the ability to learn about and help develop medical procedures. It's something that would be very difficult for a teenager nowadays with all the rules and regulations. However, if it weren't for the less restrictive nature of the medical industry 50 years ago and all those who took a chance on me, I would have never experienced a career that allowed me to help pioneer treatments and technologies to prevent and fight heart disease.

Toward the end of writing this book, my closest friend throughout all of my youth in Hillsdale, Michigan, paid me a visit. We did everything together, and when I heard he was coming for a visit, I asked him to bring any material that might be helpful for this book. He brought the 1953 Hillsdale High School yearbook, which had a copy of *Reflections*.

This publication showcased student writing at Hillsdale High School from 1952 to 1953. I was on the editorial staff of that publication and contributed two articles. I have included them to introduce the dramatic turn my writing underwent after entering the University of Michigan:

"Pes" Pains
Ted Diethrich grade 12

Seven inches, twelve inches, size eight, size thirteen, too loose, too tight, too long, too short…are the cries of the American women when describing a foot condition either with or without a shoe. Now, since I am neither a medical doctor, a chiropodist, nor a cobbler, my advice on the subject lacks sound foundation; therefore, I propose to relate only my theory on "Pes" Pains. And if, perchance, a reader should happen to agree with my hypothesis, I will not only be delighted, but might also have the courage to work toward a PhD in chiropody.

First, let us discuss the causes of soreness in the lower extremities of the body. In ancient China, the feet of small girls were tightly wrapped, thus hindering their proper development and growth. Now we laugh at such an absurd practice, but in reality the fairer sex follows the same procedure today, with a few variations of course. This catastrophe occurs about the of age of fourteen, when girls find they have reached the age that requires more clothes, more primping and naturally, high heels. It is the latter item that is the destructive demon.

As I have already remarked, my authority on the subject is limited, and the fact that I am a male further hinders my qualifications to analyze this problem. Nevertheless, from my acute observations, I have been able to conclude these important facts about elevated shoes. It is not enough that women want to remove their heels from the same plane as their toes; but at the same time they desire a shoe wide enough for only four-fifths of the toes. The other fifth is to be jammed in, thus producing the snug feeling. Conclusion: this shoe is the main cause of sore feet, and the varying types of shoes, namely the height of the heel, determine the degree of distress.

With this important conclusion determined, we are prepared to investigate the effects the said shoes produce on the ordinary foot. Without a doubt, everyone is familiar with the common ailments… corns, blisters and bunions; so I shall refrain from discussing them and proceed to more uncommon effects.

The chief distress comes from the tourniquet effect produced by the shoe. Before the application of this monster, the foot has a natural color; the toes are soft and pink; and the circulation is adequate. The change that occurs during a few hours of poor circulation is unbelievable.

When the shoe is pried off the natural color has been replaced by a deep blue; the pink toes have also taken on a bluish cast; and as for circulation, the veins are so compressed that the blood goes no further than the ankle.

The above fact sounds incredible, but actually the seriousness is very minute compared to the difficulty encountered in the bones. In six months, a normal well-developed foot becomes a cramped up, distorted looking object that only its owner could recognize this part of the human body. The inevitable outcome is costly x-rays, continual foot treatment, and flat-soled shoes. From this short, yet quite thorough dissertation, one can readily see the seriousness of the feminine foot condition today. It would certainly seem that women, noted for their wise judgment, would have taken a lesson from the Chinese and abandoned the torture of "Pes" pains with the abolishment of the high heel and narrow shoe.

American-style
Ted Diethrich grade 12

Most people in the professional field
Do not to this Temptation yield
To the high sophisticated class it's trite,
And most intelligentsia would say they're right.
All children, especially young, seem to love it.
All teachers, both young and old, seem to hate it.
If you know, tell me, what is it?
We've been too long mum.
The subject is gum!

There's a question in my mind of whether gum chewing is a universal pastime; however, there's little doubt about its use in the United States. Wherever we go or whatever we do we can be assured of seeing and feeling gum. I use the word feeling discriminately; for I presume that you, as I, have had the experience of sitting down in a restaurant and accidentally feeling beneath the table. What did you find? Gum, American-style!

A person ignorant of the fact that gum is to be chewed might possibly think its use is primarily to hold the stuffing in theater seats, or to prevent slipping on the floor, or better yet to prevent the combing of boys and girls hair. And of course in any discussion of gum, we should not forget its use as a solder behind the ear.

Actually there is some fallacy in the use of gum mentioned above, for its real purpose is to keep the teeth clean, white and without cavities "so the manufacturers say"; to use after eating onions, thus preventing the loss of friends; and finally, to relax or stiffen the jaw muscles, whichever the case may be.

From my observations I have come to the conclusion that there are four types of gum chewers. The first, and probably the least annoying, is the dormant gum chewer. He holds his gum in abeyance, either under his tongue, on the roof of his mouth, or plastered on his teeth somewhere. He has no definite pattern to his chewing, and often it may be hard to detect the presence of any gum in his mouth.

One will have no difficulty in the second case, however, for though his lips are tightly closed, his jaws move as rapidly as a secondhand of a clock. The one consolation is that since the lips are closed, we are spared from any sound.

This, unfortunately, is not the pattern of our next example. No, he is not content unless his teeth are apart, jaws widely spread, and he is making a considerable amount of smacking noise. This type of gum chewer is obnoxious; for his jaws are constantly chunking in somewhat of a rhythmic motion... much like the tick of a metronome. I give this person my condolences, but his jaws must get terribly tired. The fourth member of this union is the half and half chewer. He, like none of the other, makes sure he gets his money's worth. While he chews part of the gum, the other half is stretched a quarter way across the room, and this statement is only slight exaggeration. With the strands of sticky gum wrapped artistically around his finger, and a sizable wad in his mouth, this person is really prepared to enjoy himself.

Possibly before we close this discussion, it would be well to distinguish the two categories of gum chewers in relation to time. First, there is the assiduous chewer who is never without a piece of gum in his mouth. I am quite apathetic for this person's jaws; for certainly they must have become immune to soreness. The other person is the one who chews at regular intervals, such as after meals, garlic, or before bedtime.

Well, it seems that we have had a paper on gum, where it is found, for what and when it is used. Other subjects might make better reading, but it is wise to know about the pastimes of Americans. And before I put the finish on this piece, let me say that the male sex is no more guilty of the facts previously related than the females. In fact, women are the best examples of poor gum chewers.

After founding the Arizona Heart Institute in 1971, carrying out the first live televised heart surgery in 1983, performing the first heart transplant in Phoenix in 1984, and also performing Arizona's first heart and lung transplant in 1985, I'd experienced severe backlash for my methods and success, as well as international acclaim.

Today, I am the Medical Director of the Arizona Heart Foundation, a separate non-profit organization founded in 1971. I write this life story to share my journey with friends and family, former and current colleagues, students wanting a different perspective of the medical industry, or just an audience interested in a true story that combines historical advancements, a look into the operating room through my eyes, and even a little bit of scandal. I hope it shows that if you are passionate about your interests, you can change the course of history with hard work and dedication.

This book is a ride through my professional and personal life, threaded with stories that may fascinate or appall. From assisting with my first surgery at the age of sixteen to a career filled with world-renowned surgical advancements, a love for music, and even some encounters with the "Medical Mafia," this is my serendipitous life.

Introduction

As I slipped down the stairs from my room, the sun was just rising. Through the front door's window, I could see that a beautiful blanket of snow had fallen during the night at our home in Hillsdale, Michigan; at least six inches of the white powdery stuff. I was surprised that the Christmas tree lights were already twinkling, although I shouldn't have been.

My mother, Nina Amanda Kilgore, was the matriarch of the family and certainly in charge of every aspect of Christmas week, from cooking and baking to supervising the tree decorations.

Most important, she reveled in constantly running the vacuum cleaner over the red carpet that covered the entire first floor. For some reason, that carpet attracted every piece of lint in the air.

Mom had no doubt been up for more than two hours with early morning preparations. The tree looked beautiful, much more brilliant than the trees most have today. Behind every bulb there was a carefully placed mirror-like reflector, causing

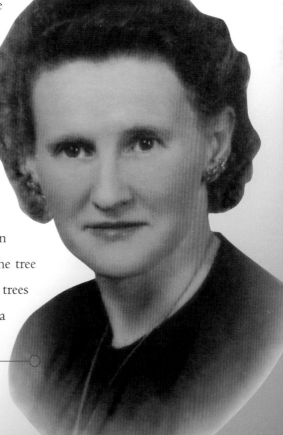

My mother, Nurse Nina Amanda Kilgore.

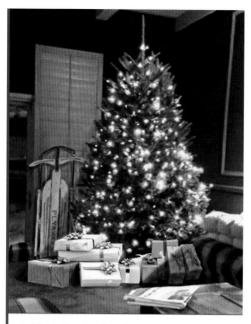

Behind the family Christmas tree was my special present.

each and every tree branch to glisten, and a magnificent star adorned the top.

Although we had cousins, nieces, aunts, uncles, and grandparents who had gathered from various parts of the state and beyond, no one was in sight. I was sure my mom was in the kitchen, but none of that mattered. My eyes scanned across the multitude of brightly wrapped presents, and the large pile made it obvious that there was more than one or two for everyone.

Then I spotted it directly behind the tree, against the angle of the wall. The only present I had requested from Santa via letter. My heart was in my throat; I had waited so long for this moment. It was magnificent and shiny as it reflected the tree's lights, and the glistening smooth wood contrasted with the red metal components.

There it was: my flexible Red Flyer sled, poised to meet the challenge of our overnight gift from the clouds. Mom appeared from the kitchen, sharing my excitement, and helped me free my trophy from the multitude of other presents.

Holiday ritual ensued. Everyone sipped coffee and hot chocolate as the youngest acted as Santa's elf, dispensing the goodies throughout the family. After that we sat down to a hearty breakfast, one surely not approved on my current health program. However, all of the ritual activities could not be over fast enough for me. There was only one thing on my mind: the sled.

Finally it came time when I could approach Uncle Ken, who clearly shared my excitement in my new present. He quickly accepted my offer for a sled race, and we donned our snow clothes and marched up the street together with the Red Flyer. Hill Street was perfect for sledding; it originated almost at my back door and

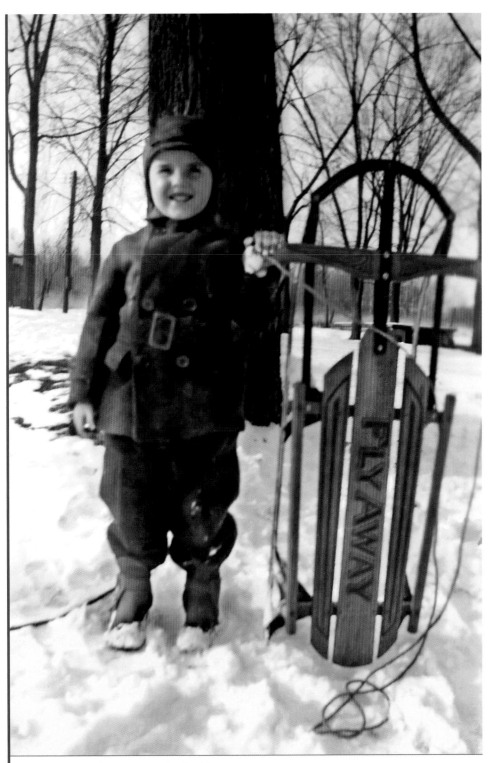

Waiting for Uncle Ken to begin the big race.

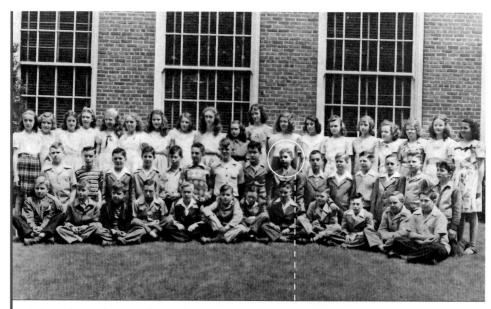

Sixth grade graduation photo. There was no dress code imposed, but it is obvious that a necktie culture existed, championed by my parents, which carried through to high school graduation and beyond. I am in the middle row, seventh from the right.

coursed downward past Cold Springs Park, where we skated and played hockey. Then it followed up the incline to cross the railroad tracks, ending with a really fast downhill run.

Of course there was no doubt who would use which sled. Uncle Ken picked the one that probably generated similar excitement some years before. I climbed on the new Flyer, and we began the race down Hill Street to the railroad crossing. The snow was just right for speed.

We whizzed past the pond at Cold Springs, and I had the lead over my uncle. Suddenly, as I crossed the railroad tracks, I hit a snow embankment on the left and lost control. The Flyer flew into the air, propelling me into a snowdrift. No pain, just shame. Snow was crusted all over my face and body. Uncle Ken was quick to the rescue. As he peered to look for an injured Ted, I muttered, "Uncle Ken, I was made for work, not play."

This is the story of that work and then some.

And it's been quite a ride!

SLED

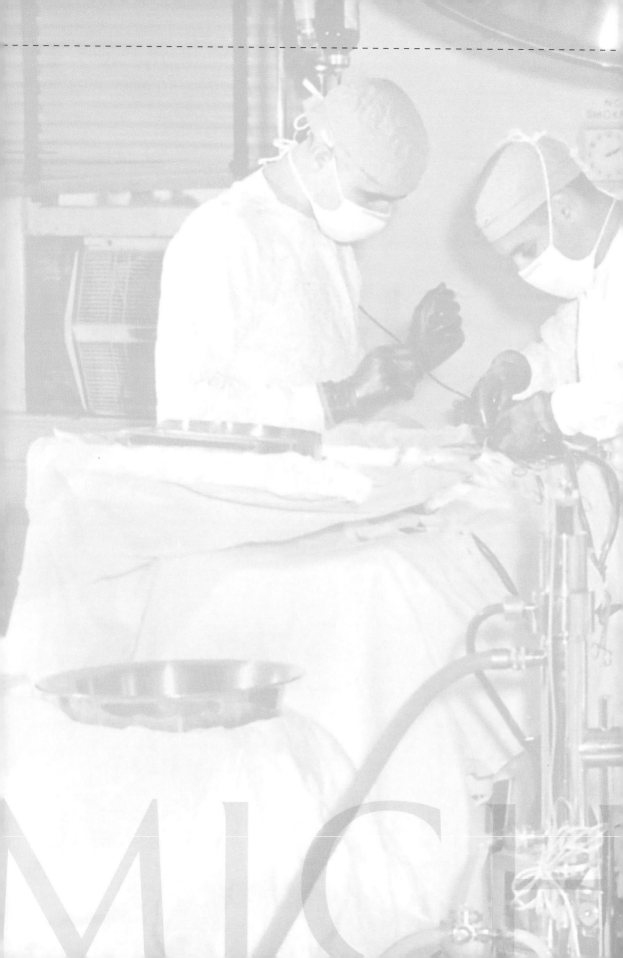

MICHIGAN

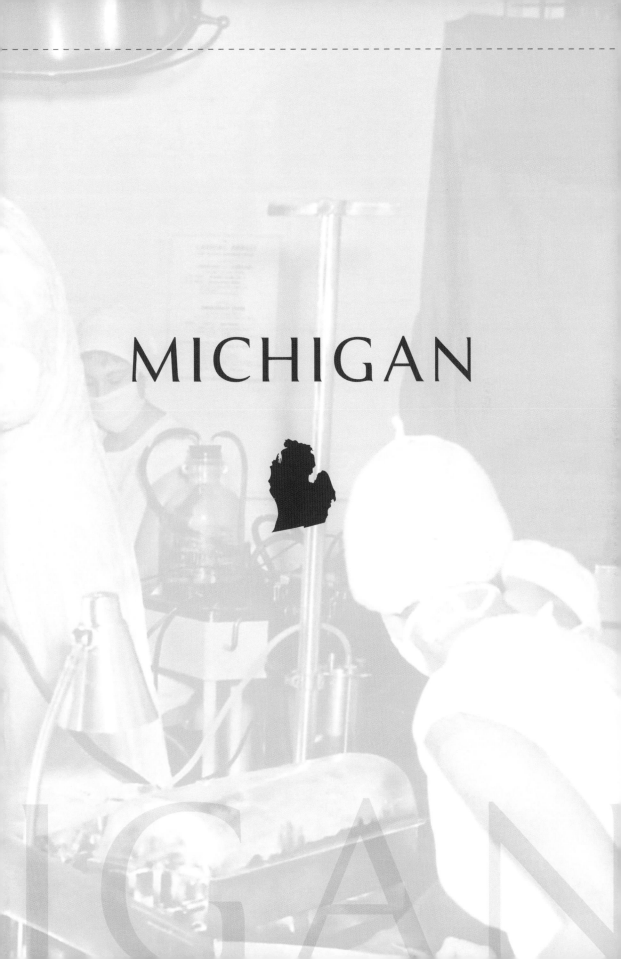

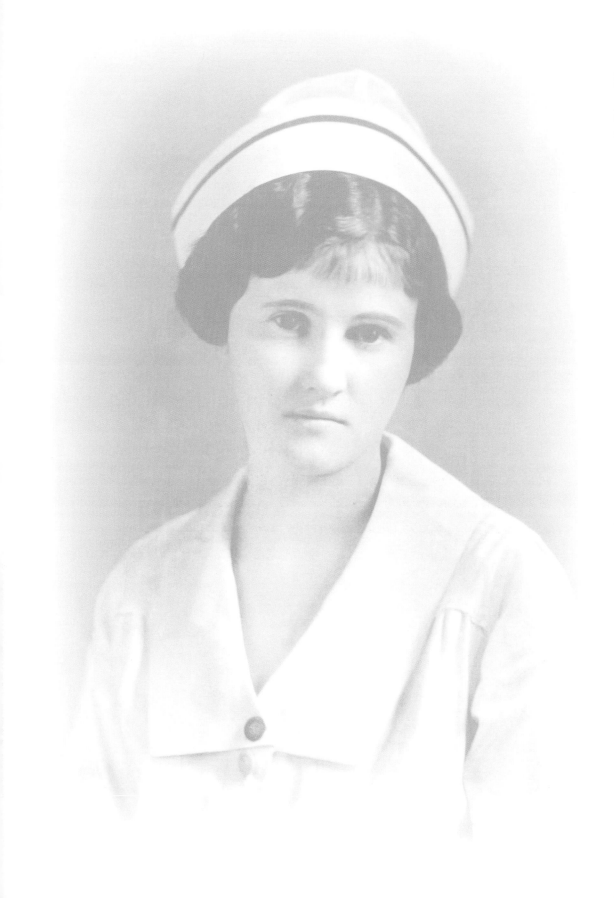

1

The Beginning,
An Orderly Fib at Fifteen

Hillsdale was a small town in southern Michigan, surrounded by several towns that were even less populated. While it was locally known as the hub for the "world's most famous" county fair each fall, Hillsdale was also the county seat, ideally placed for a central medical facility serving the residents.

Hillsdale Community Hospital was a shining star. Not only was the physical plant very modern for its time, it also provided excellent care and the best surgical services for 50 miles around. When my mother graduated from Flower Hospital in Toledo, Ohio, she specialized in operating room nursing. After several years and two sons, she decided to return to her nursing career and began to provide private duty care at the Hillsdale Hospital.

People have always asked me when and why I decided to become a doctor, and the answer is clearly related to my experience at the hospital with my mother.

When I was free from school activities and sports, I'd sit next to her, watching and listening to the specialized care she provided. In those days, usually the very ill

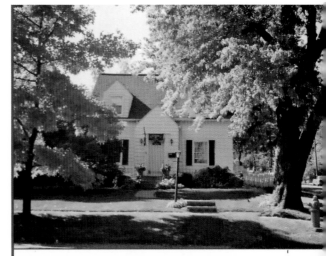

My family home in Hillsdale, Michigan.
Left: My mother, Nina Amanda Kilgore, RN.

patients were enclosed within an oxygen tent. Most people today have never even heard of those. It was a very special opportunity for a young boy to be able to witness that high level of patient care and concern from a nurse.

The most significant part, though, was that I could have the many questions swirling in my head answered by my own mother. It was clear in those very early days that I was headed toward medicine in some way, but as a student in high school, I had a full agenda.

Academics were high priority, but my life was filled with extracurricular activities, such as being president of student council, editor of the Twin Towers (the school paper), band, orchestra, state competitions, and especially sports. But I was drawn like a magnet to the community hospital. Unbelievably, I secured a job as an orderly at the age of 15. I actually had to fib because the minimum age for employment was 16. But it was the most important fib I ever told because it opened extraordinary experiences that influenced many of my future medical pursuits.

The orderly's main responsibility was to wheel the patient from the ward to the operating room and execute the reverse when the procedure was completed. Fortunately for me, something else special happened. My mother decided to transfer from special duty medical nursing to an operating room nurse

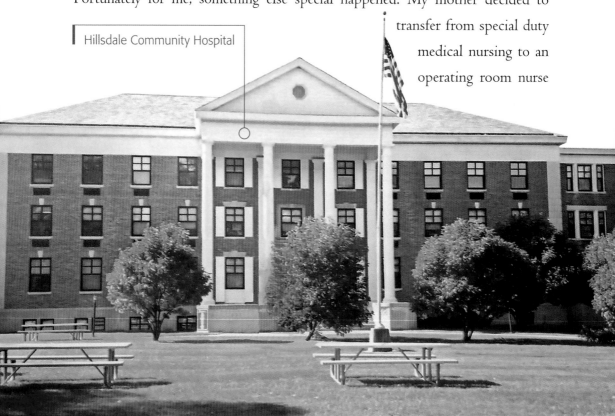

Hillsdale Community Hospital

position. There was a small staff and only two operating rooms, which meant that whenever I wasn't busy moving patients, I could stand near the anesthetist and observe the operative procedures. The surgeons were quite eager to point out what they were doing, even to a 15-year-old high school student. And later on in the evening at home, my mom would patiently answer my myriad of questions.

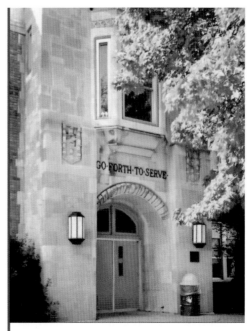

The high school motto was "Enter to Learn, Go Forth to Serve." This is alluded to in my graduation speech to the Hillsdale class of 1974 (see Chapter 44).

Many years later, shortly after I performed the first open-heart operation on national live television, I received a kind letter from Dr. Fraser Mattson, the Chief of Surgery at the Hillsdale Hospital. He congratulated me on the televised case explaining that I, as a high school student, had seen him perform a hernia repair many years before. It was actually the first one I ever observed, and now he had seen me performing a triple coronary artery bypass procedure, the first one he had ever witnessed.

Hillsdale was one of the counties hit heaviest with the polio epidemic. Almost on a weekly basis, a patient was transferred from Hillsdale to Ann Arbor, Michigan, for treatment at the University Hospital, usually for use of the "iron lung" to support respiratory failure. Under ideal conditions, a nurse or even a doctor would accompany the patient in the ambulance for the transfer; sometimes I rode with them.

One evening my mother said there was a transfer scheduled for the next day, but nobody was available to ride with the patient and they wanted me to go. However, the next afternoon I was supposed to compete in a track meet in Adrian, Michigan. I called my coach and said I couldn't make the track meet because I had to work. He was furious. My dad supported my decision in spite of his athletic influence on me.

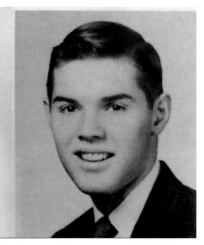

EDWARD DIETHRICH
Class Officer 2-3, Hi-Y 2-3-4, Latin Club
1-2, Senior Band 1-2-3-4, Orchestra 3-4,
Officer 3-4, H-Club 1-2-3-4, Student Council 2-3, Basketball: Reserve 2, Varsity 3-4,
Football: Reserve 1-2, Varsity 3-4, Track
1-2.

In addition to a full schedule, time was still squeezed in for an active hospital experience while in high school.

When I ran into the coach early the next day in the school hallway, he said if I failed to run that afternoon I would have to forfeit my varsity letter in track. It meant I would not letter in three major sports, which was my athletic goal. I had a hard decision to make, but it would not be the last time that sports and medicine would simultaneously occupy my life.

After school that day, I found myself in the ambulance. The patient was a young child, obviously having trouble breathing despite the oxygen. Keep in mind that none of the high-tech equipment used today was invented yet. My duty was to take the boy's pulse and report his condition to the ambulance driver; there was not really much else to do. The polio victims were desperate, and until they reached the iron lung, their condition was perilous. Such was this case.

We were not more than forty-five minutes underway when his pulse faded and the labored respirations ceased. I reported the child's condition to the driver, and we immediately headed back to Hillsdale.

That would not be the last time a victim of polio would be lost in transit. However, it was my first experience with human death outside the hospital, without a nurse such as my mother to support me. It was not a great day. I had witnessed a young boy dying, and let my coach and fellow track mates down in the competition.

It wasn't until much later I learned my work would often present situations with conflicting decisions. At graduation, Coach Inman presented me with all three letters. With tearful eyes, I shook his hand with a grateful thank you.

Between athletics, music, and schoolwork, I had limited time for much else. However, Saturdays were usually free for me to go to the operating room and observe the procedures. Those days were special because the general practitioners from all over the county would come to perform their more minor surgical procedures. The most common was a tonsillectomy and adenoidectomy (also called a "T&A"), which was almost a required operation for every child in those days. The second most common procedure was a vasectomy, a procedure to create male sterilization, and it was the specialty of one of the general surgeons from North Adams.

The operating room seen so frequently on television today shows much glitz and glamour, but behind the scenes it is very different. Washing, checking, and sterilizing the instruments from the various operations is a big job, and the Saturday morning general practitioner provided a lot of work for my mother and other nurses; there were no techs in those days. It was the perfect setting to learn the names and use for each of the instruments as they were going through the cleaning process. Mom would wash the instrument, declaring, "Hemostat, used to clamp vessels and stop bleeding." Then she would pass it on to me for drying, and I had to restate the name and function: "Hemostat, to clamp vessels and stop the bleeding." This was repeated over and over again for just one instrument, and there must have been 50 hemostats in every instrument tray. Then the Alice clamps, Babcock clamps, and even Halstead retractors followed.

At the time it never occurred to me that the instruments were probably named after the famous surgeons who had invented them, much like I did later in life with the Sternal Saw and Coronary Kit. In fact, many years later,

My father, Thurman Clarence, "T.C." Diethrich, also known as "Bud."

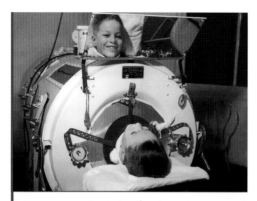

A young patient in the Iron Lung—most commonly used for polio victims with respiratory failure.

while standing in the operating room in Milan, Italy, I heard the surgeon call for the Diethrich circumflex scissors. A special feeling of pride came over me; I appreciated that recognition.

During the days of naming instruments, I saw Dr. Mattson use the Badgley nail to put a fractured hip back together. It was an amazing procedure. The bone and joint devices were distinctly different from the other general surgery instruments, as were the operative procedures themselves. But the real significance of the Badgley procedure would not be apparent to me until later on, during my second hospital job.

The county surgeons operated with the help of only one nurse. The anesthesia was open drop ether, where at times I believe the anesthetist received more anesthesia than the patient. There seemed to always be the need for another pair of hands to retract or assist with the suckers to remove blood, particularly in the T&A procedure. Who better to help than the son of the head nurse who was also a young "student"?

Then one Saturday morning, an epiphany occurred. The North Adam's surgeon was doing a vasectomy and having trouble locating the vas deferens, the tube that connects the testicle to deliver sperm. Maybe my fingers were more nimble or eyesight more acute, but it turned out to be my very first vasectomy. Of course, these types of experiences could not exist today, and this book is filled with them, but they no doubt shaped my attitude for the future of my work.

Hillsdale Community Hospital and Nina Amanda Kilgore Diethrich, my mother/nurse/teacher, were a real ride for a young boy, but on high school graduation day, I tossed my cap in the air with the rest of my classmates and left immediately for the University of Michigan. I never really appreciated how lucky I was as a young kid from the little town of Hillsdale, armed with more medical knowledge than I realized. And I had no idea where life's paths would lead me.

2

A Mission Not So Impossible

It might seem as though I was more anxious to leave Hillsdale than my schoolmates, but my life's mission officially began with high school graduation. The first task was getting to Ann Arbor and settling into college life as rapidly as possible.

I knew in spite of my excellent preparation, the University of Michigan would be an academic challenge, especially in the premedical school curriculum. I wanted to get a jump start by taking freshman English and biology, as I thought summer school would give me more time for studying.

That was a complete miscalculation, since the second and third priorities for getting to Ann Arbor turned out to be very time-consuming.

One of those top priorities was finding a way to support the costs of college. I had received a scholarship to cover tuition, but in those days that was only a tiny component of the annual expenses. So, I needed a good job that could accommodate my school requirements.

It's amazing how few job skills students in those days had after twelve

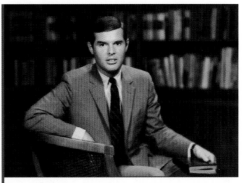

Entering the freshman class at the University of Michigan. I was a serious student with my mind clearly set on becoming a doctor.

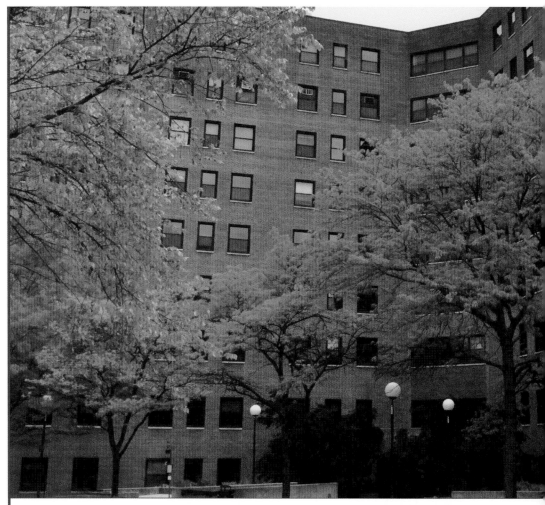

Entrance to the original St. Joseph's Hospital in Ann Arbor, Michigan—my home for nine years as well as the site of the dog lab where I spent hours working on investigative projects.

years of education, but maybe it's no different today. Regardless, I did have the differentiating experience of my high school hospital work. It seemed logical to apply for a job as an operating room orderly at St. Joseph's Mercy Hospital, the large general hospital in Ann Arbor that was affiliated with the university. I wasted no time.

After checking into my summer dorm, East Quad, and picking up my course schedule, I walked to the corner of Catherine and Ingalls streets and directly through the front door of St. Joe's. It was an important first step into my future,

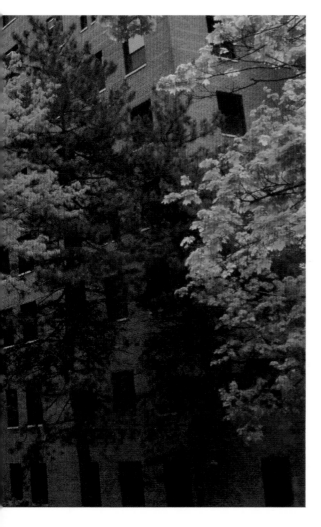

and I would continue to walk through those doors for many years to come.

"May I help you, sir?" the receptionist asked, looking up at me.

"Yes, I would like to meet the supervisor of the operating rooms to inquire about an orderly position," I replied.

"Take the elevator directly behind you to the second floor, turn right, and you will be there."

"Thank you, ma'am."

Can you imagine how that conversation would sound today?

"You will have to go downstairs to the Department of Human Resources. Fill out ten to twelve pages of information, and make an appointment to return to be interviewed by one of the HR Supervisors. I am not sure that department is open today..."

I could feel the slight moisture on my fingers as I pushed the second floor elevator button, but it was nothing compared to the full-blown, perspiration-inducing experience I was about to witness. As I stepped off the elevator, I easily spotted an OR nurse because of her attire.

"Excuse me, could you direct me to the OR Director's office?" I inquired.

"You are there, next door on the left," replied the nurse hurriedly.

"Thank you." I was very nervous, but these people seemed extremely nice. Maybe it would be a pleasant place for me to work? Following the instructions, I gave a gentle knock on the first door on the left and waited until I heard a seemingly emotionless "come in."

Upon opening the door, the lack of vocal expression and the visual of the person behind it instantly caused panic to well up within me.

Sitting behind a sterile-looking desk was a nun in a white habit. The only thing whiter in the room was her complexion. Pale, no smile, expressionless.

In order to understand my reaction, one has to know I was raised Presbyterian. And while there was an active Catholic community in Hillsdale, it was not a part of my upbringing. The nuns I had encountered were clothed in black habits, so this was truly a cultural experience; just one of many I would experience during my Michigan days.

She motioned to the chair in front of me. "Sit down," she said in a monotone voice. "What do you want to see me about?"

I sat down and tried to appear confident and relaxed, but I did not even know how to address her. Director, Sister, Supervisor? I was sure it was not Miss, Mrs, or Madame, so I used none of those.

Luckily, she came to my rescue. "I am Sister Mary Xavier, the operating room supervisor here at St. Joseph's Hospital. I understand you are looking for work. Your name is?"

I quickly responded, "Ted Diethrich."

"And what is it you are aspiring for your career?"

"I want to become a doctor, and I need a job to help support my studies," I said in one long exhale.

"And your work experience…?" she prompted. Suddenly it was easier. I could talk about my mother, the operating room experience in Hillsdale, my orderly duties. My confidence level increased, and my skin began to dry.

"When are you available to work?"

"My last class ends each day at 2 p.m."

"Well report here Monday at 3 p.m."

That was it, short and to the point. I got the job! So much for preferential treatment based on religious beliefs! I was already on my way for the next unbelievable ride.

Now it was time to focus on my second summer priority: my goal to join the Michigan Marching Band. I knew that passing and running on the Michigan football field was beyond my skill level, but playing the trumpet was a distinct possibility. Competition for the then all male, 140-member band was tough, but I had a superb background and felt as though all I needed were some private lessons during summer school.

So, I made arrangements for daily one-hour sessions in between my two school lessons. The effort was well worth it, and on opening football Saturday I found myself on the field. It was the thrill of a lifetime to march through the tunnel and then onto the 50-yard line at 160 beats-per-minute, the stadium roaring as we played the famous "Hail to the Victors" tradition.

My first day of work at St. Joseph's turned out to be an experience that would profoundly influence the future of my professional career. When I arrived in the operating room and changed clothes in preparation for my orderly duties, I reported back to Sister Xavier's office as she had directed. She introduced me to Peggy Early, a pretty young nurse with a friendly smile.

"Mr. Diethrich, I will take you to operating Room #4 where Dr. Badgley is finishing a hip-pinning operation," she explained.

What? The same "Dr. Badgley" procedure I had witnessed in Hillsdale months before, performed by Dr. Mattson? The excitement was almost uncontrollable. We arrived at the room, and I noted the stretcher parked outside the doors. I took a position next to it in preparation for transporting the patient to the recovery room.

To my amazement, Miss Early handed me an OR cap and mask and directed me to the scrub sink. "Scrub up and go into the room. You will replace the scrub nurse who is going off duty in ten minutes." From drying and naming instruments in a community hospital 90 miles away to scrubbing for one of the world's most famous orthopedic surgeons—could this really be happening to me? My initial encounter with Sister Xavier must have set a protocol for me.

I didn't say a word. I just proceeded into the operating room, introduced myself to the scrub and circulation nurses, put on my OR gown and gloves, and took my

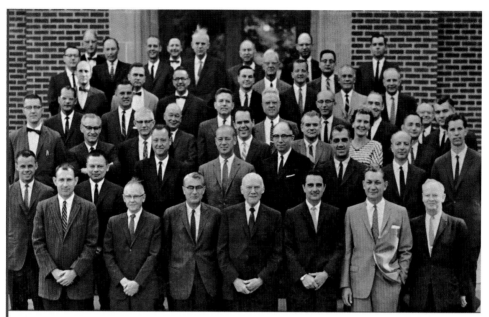

The surgical staff of St. Joe's, all with University of Michigan faculty appointments.

position at the operating table, directly next to Dr. Badgley's left elbow. Fortunately for me, the procedure was about completed and the closure was not complicated. All went well, and I was thrilled with both the experience and the opportunity. I must confess, I never told any of the operating room personnel that I was hired as an orderly.

From that day until I graduated from medical school and started my internship, I had a scrub nurse position at St. Joe's, although it was mostly due to the fact that they didn't have techs in those days. I was also often on the call schedule, which was even better because the pay was much higher and I could fit work into my other activities and school preparations.

This was a fortunate job opportunity, but in reality it became invaluable to my career progress. All of the most important surgeons at the University of Michigan Medical School and Hospital also had practices at St. Joe's. Professor Badgley in orthopedics, as an example, but the same held true for neuro, thoracic, general, and ear, nose and throat (ENT) surgery. In fact, the dean of the medical school practiced his ENT specialty three days a week. I met all of these superstars and worked side-by-side with them as a premedical student and later as a medical student. Most of them knew me by my first name, and I took advantage of every opportunity to indulge in conversations between the operations.

One of these specialists became not only a close friend, but also initiated my further interest in research and biomedical engineering. Dr. Clarence Crook, a general surgeon, was working one evening a week in his homemade dog lab located in the hospital basement.

His main interest was blood vessels, and he had fabricated tubes that could be sutured into place to repair diseased arteries. (It's important to remember that at the time there were no commercial grafts as we know them today, but much more on that later.)

The dog lab was a small room equipped with all used or rejected supplies from the operating room, and the dogs were strays donated for research purposes. I took advantage of every opportunity to work with Dr. Crook because he was actually teaching me to operate, tie knots, sew in grafts, and close incisions, among many other things.

It wasn't long until I became a fixture in the lab, and conditions gradually improved, mostly because of what I could "confiscate" from the human operating room three floors up.

Much later we expanded the lab to outside the hospital, and by that time I had become very good friends with the hospital administrator, Sister Mary Leonette.

In fact, my daughter was named Mary Lynne after this nun. I convinced Sister Leonette we could construct a very nice laboratory in the garage outside the back door where the nuns parked their cars. We built two concrete wall pens directly next to where the "nun mobiles" parked. It really was a first-class lab by standards of those days, but of course it would not pass muster by today's regulations. We operated

Dr. Clarence Crook—an early mentor offering a unique opportunity for me in the basement dog lab.

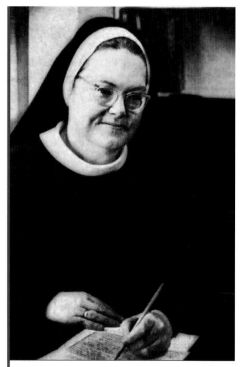

Sister Mary Leonette, at times foe, but in the end a true friend.

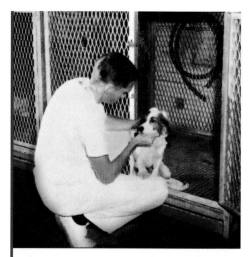

The recovering patient back in his pen, which was not nearly as comfortable as the backseat of the nun mobile.

on Wednesday evenings and Saturdays, time permitting.

All was well until my phone rang early one Sunday morning with a very irritated Sister Mary Leonette on the other end of the line.

"Mr. Diethrich, one of your dogs is in the rear seat of our car, and we are late for church!"

I raced to the lab, but by the time I arrived the recovering animal was back in his pen. The perpetrator who pulled that stunt was never identified, but it took me months to get back on the good side of Sister Mary Leonette. Our laboratory work continued and, even as a premedical student, my potential surgical skills were starting to gain recognition by the attending staff.

3

Flying Through the
University of Michigan

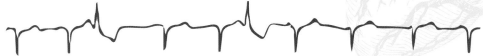

My undergraduate days were gone in a flash. In just three years, I completed six semesters of seventeen to eighteen credit hours each and three consecutive sessions of summer school. My studies were also coupled with regular hospital work, research, enjoyment of the band, and fraternity life.

The day after college graduation, my high school sweetheart, Gloria Baldwin, and I were married. She had graduated from the Ypsilanti Teachers College (now known as Eastern Michigan University) with a major in special education. Very conveniently, she had secured a position in the hospital school at the University Hospital and later in my training we would even pass each other in the pediatric wards.

I applied only to the University of Michigan Medical School, and fortunately I was accepted in June 1956. Not with the highest grade point average I must say, but I had been a busy lad. The only downside to entering medical school was the necessity to drop the band. There was just not enough time with all the laboratory courses.

I had only been in medical school a few months when I had a phone call from my Uncle Mart in Hillsdale. He informed me that my mother was very ill and that I should come home immediately. Gloria and I left that afternoon and drove directly to the Hillsdale Hospital where I had worked while in high school.

We met Uncle Mart and he led us to a room on the second floor. There was a bed with an oxygen tent identical to the one my mother worked with when doing private nursing and I sat next to her asking questions. The tent was moist, making it hard to see inside. I pulled the zipper on the panel and peered inside. Mom was asleep, breathing heavily. I noted that the head of the bed was in an erect position. I leaned forward to kiss her on the forehead and she suddenly opened her eyes. She looked at me and in a frail voice said, "Ted, what are you doing here?" She went back to sleep. I closed the panel zipper and turned to be greeted by her internal medicine physician, Dr. Strom, who had cared for our family many years. He sat down next to me. I could tell by his facial expression this was not good news.

"Your mother is in severe congestive heart failure. Two of her valves are not working and in spite of the medications and oxygen, I don't think she can survive much longer."

No one could have anticipated that forty years later these valves could be replaced with new ones without use of the heart-lung machines or the need for incisions. I opened the oxygen panel again, held mom's hand, kissed her forehead, and said goodbye. We buried her three days later in Northern Ohio next to the Kilgore kin. Unfortunately, Mom never had the opportunity to appreciate her influence in the early days when she would quiz her son as he dried the surgical instruments and named them repeatedly. She would be so proud to know he went on to become a successful cardiovascular surgeon.

My father died at age 92 probably due to the ramifications of years of smoking at least a couple of packs of Lucky Strikes per day. I never had a cigarette on my lips.

An interesting side story about Uncle Mart, which relates directly to the selection of our publisher for *SLED*. My father, after leaving teaching and coaching at Howe Military School in Indiana moved to Hillsdale, Michigan, and started Bud's Hamburger Shop. It was so successful he expanded to Defiance, Ohio, and opened a second Bud's.

Uncle Mart became involved since he had family nearby in Ohio. When I was searching for a publisher, which was a pretty exhausting task, I came across Orange

Frazer Press located in Wilmington, Ohio. When I contacted them and spoke to Marcy Hawley, the publisher, I inquired about where Wilmington was located in Ohio. She answered it was far south of Defiance.

I asked her if she knew of Bud's Hamburger Shop, fully aware that it had certainly been gone for years. It did not matter. The fact that it had been there and my family was a part of it was good enough for me and the deal was closed. Can you believe it? Over a hamburger.

As a freshman in medical school in Ann Arbor, we did not have much extra time to explore the nearby "Big City" of Detroit, which was about an hour away. However, there was the occasional dinner, and more important, the occasional invitation to famous physician lectures by the sponsoring company. It was at one of these where I saw my first live telecast of Professor Charles Bailey from Philadelphia performing a coronary endarterectomy. Even at that early stage I was fascinated by the audiovisual component of surgery.

What turned out to be critical for my career path was not Detroit per se, but what surrounded it. The big three—Ford, GM and Chrysler—had their main assembly lines pushing out automobiles by the hundreds. What most people did *not* appreciate were the back resources to the lines: the small "tool and dye" shops sprawled out in towns and suburbs around the metropolis and state. These were responsible for many of the factory parts that ultimately ended up in the finished product: the automobile. This was a huge and critical industry to our country. Our location in Ann Arbor was truly ideal because the instrumentation for automobiles and the medical industry were growing at the same time.

As our surgical science advanced, my work in the dog lab spurred an ever-increasing interest in the equipment that was going to be required. Bob Richardson, a fellow medical student, and I worked to develop a device that would temporarily bypass around an artery while it was being repaired, something that Dr. Crook and I had explored. We called this new device a shunt clamp: *shunt*, because its function was to bypass, or shunt, blood during repair, and *clamp* because its mechanism temporarily clamped into the artery.

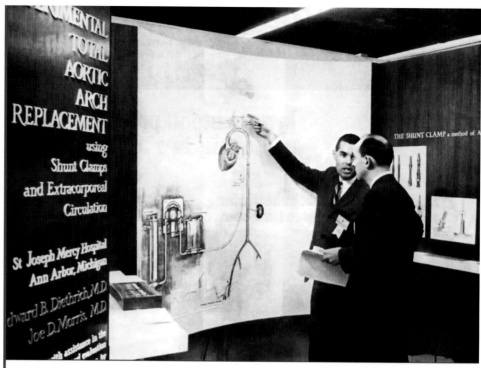

Exhibit in San Francisco of the shunt clamps we developed as medical students.

When it comes to serendipitous events, this one was really significant.

During this time, we had moved to a house in a cul-de-sac with multiple neighbors. Directly east of us next door was Dick Sarns, who ultimately became my partner in the Sarns Company. Beyond that house were several engineers who worked in those tool and dye shops near Ann Arbor.

Our homemade shunt clamp model was extremely crude, but as I met more of my engineering neighbors, it became apparent that I was in the middle of a great resource pool for the exact technology I needed. One of the major obstacles in complex vascular surgery, such as the treatment of aneurysms, was the need to temporarily interrupt the circulation to vital organs like the kidneys, brain, and spinal cord. The idea of the shunt clamp originated to solve a problem of interrupted circulation during the repair of these arterial defects. There was no way to create an aneurysm in the laboratory animals at that time, but the insertion of two shunt clamps with a connecting conduit could be tested nonetheless.

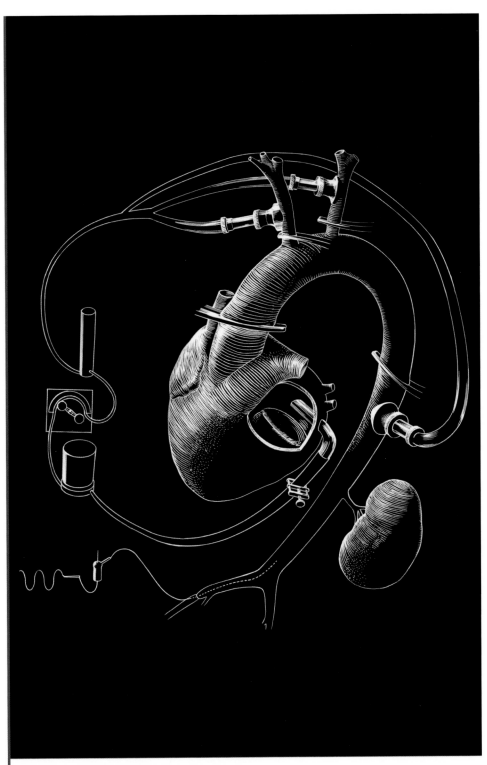

Drawing showing the use of the shunt clamp.

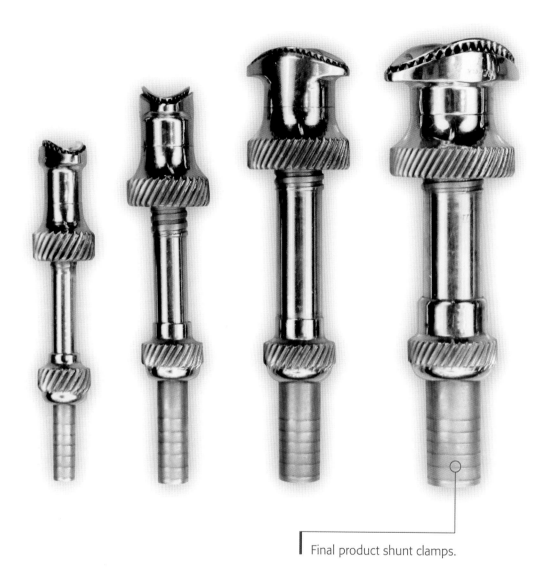

Final product shunt clamps.

Our industry partners would soon transform our crude prototype device into an instrument with a high level of perfection and sophistication.

At least twice a week we were in the laboratory, perfecting the operative techniques on our canine friends. After both the clinical and laboratory work were completed each Saturday, I went to the farm where Ed directed the farm facilities for recovering research animals for the University. At any given time there were twenty to thirty of my animals in the recuperative phase. We would make rounds together, check the incisions, and document any unusual or adverse observations.

In order to expand the engineering community, I set up an open forum once a month in the St. Joseph's Hospital auditorium. Word got out very quickly that doctors needed engineers to help save patients' lives. It was almost contagious, and before long it was not uncommon to have thirty to forty engineers present at the meetings.

It was a simple format: I presented the technical problems we were encountering in the lab and human operating rooms, and the engineers listened and provided feedback. It was easy for me to observe these needs from my position as a scrub nurse.

A high point was the shunt clamp because it made such logical engineering sense. Dick Sarns was always present at those meetings, and we would frequently huddle in my kitchen or driveway to assess the progress of the ideas and devices.

Since the engineers were widely dispersed in their work environment, they had numerous contacts. When the shunt clamp proved to work in the laboratory, everyone was eager to talk about it. *The Detroit Free Press* even had a front-page story, complete with a picture of Bob and me holding the shunt clamp. At the time, it seemed very innocuous. My other classmates were intrigued with the story because our lab work was always during after school hours or on weekends when they were not around. Unfortunately, the praise was short-lived.

Word spread about the newspaper article and by noon we were in the dean of the medical school's office, severely reprimanded for not obtaining permission to meet the press. Like two small kids, all we could do was apologize, say we

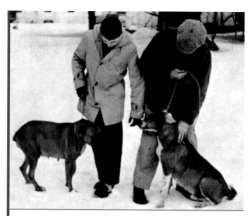

Postoperative animals, which were to be studied for long periods, were cared for at our nearby farm.

didn't know the rules, and reassure it would not happen again. That was my introduction to the media-medical connection; I would later become somewhat of an expert on this subject.

While the University was not too excited about the newspaper article, my corps of engineers was thrilled. The ability to access and control the new investigative laboratory at St. Joe's provided a unique opportunity for an aspiring young student.

I had become a good friend of Dr. Joe Morris, a professor of thoracic surgery at the University. He was very helpful and advised me on my work with total aortic arch replacement using the shunt clamps and extracorporeal circulation, which meant using a pumping system to maintain blood pressure. These investigations were extremely exciting and ended up being my introduction to the heart/lung machine.

Each year, the American College of Surgeons (ACS) held a clinical congress with a sponsored scientific exhibit session. I was convinced the shunt clamp project with total aortic arch replacement was progressing to the point of meriting a display at the ACS meeting in San Francisco in October of 1963.

I submitted an abstract for the scientific exhibit session and found myself in disbelief: I was assigned Scientific Exhibit S-33 at the 49th Annual Clinical Congress of the American College of Surgeons.

Now what had I done? Who was to build the exhibit? More important, who would *pay* for it? And lastly, we were in Ann Arbor, three-quarters of the way across the country from San Francisco!

Okay, one problem at a time. I had made a friend at the art department of the university, Jerry Hodge, through an introduction by Joe Morris. He agreed to help with the exhibit. By that time, Sister Mary Leonette had forgiven me for the dog-

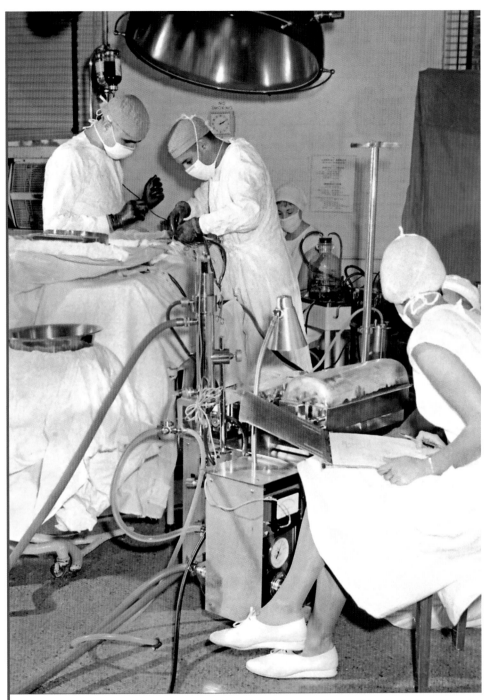

This experiment was the precursor of the clinical case performed by Dr. Robert Spetzler at Barrow's Neurological Institute where the patient was cooled with the heat exchanger (see Chapter 4). The circulation was stopped in order to permit the clipping of a large intracranial aneurysm.

in-the-back-seat-of-the-nun-mobile incident and agreed to pay the expenses. That was really quite a big deal for them!

There was one obstacle left: How would we transport the exhibit all the way across the country without breaking the budget, a budget that I had never even seen?

Every Sunday in the *Detroit Free Press,* there were a number of listings for cars available to drive from Detroit to the West Coast. It was an inexpensive way to move vehicles over a long distance. I saw such an ad and made the call.

"Yes, we have a vehicle we need delivered from Detroit to San Francisco," said the voice on the other end of the line. That was all I needed to hear, so I made the arrangements to pick the car up at the transportation headquarters in Detroit.

John Liddicoat and Jim Wessinger, two of my trusted medical student friends, joined me on the trip to Detroit. We checked in at the office, presented a driver's license, and signed the necessary forms for transfer. We then were led into the parking lot, where the attendant pointed to a vehicle. It was a brand new, white Cadillac convertible with 10 miles on the speedometer.

Can you imagine the expression on our faces, obviously muted to reduce attendant apprehension about letting some students drive that special vehicle across the country?

There was no way we could tell the transport agency that we needed a trailer hitch attachment for a rented U-Haul, one that was going to haul an exhibit 2,000 or more miles to the West Coast. We just ignored that detail altogether; so now, on to Ann Arbor with the top down. No wonder the dean was suspicious of Ted Diethrich, the medical student, corrupting two more of his pupils.

Once on campus, we executed our plan, attaching the trailer hitch and loading the exhibit. The trip from Ann Arbor to San Francisco was going to take around two days. The agency had said the car needed to be delivered in seven to nine days, which provided some leeway for bad weather, mechanical problems, or whatever else we might encounter. We figured with three drivers we could go around the clock, drop the trailer off at a friend of Jim's in San Francisco, and have plenty of time for sightseeing in our convertible. We did just that.

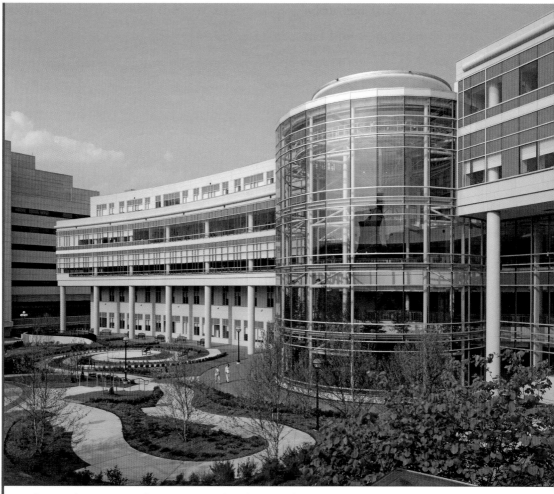

Cardiovascular Center at the University of Michigan today.

On the opening day of the exhibit, I eagerly anticipated meeting the surgeons and showing our work. I had just finished talking to one eager visitor at our table, when I turned and saw none other than Dr. Denton Cooley viewing our material. I had never met him, but had seen him talk at several meetings.

I introduced myself and asked if he had any questions. He commented that the technique seemed to have promise. Never did I think that one day I would be a resident working with such a famous surgeon.

Back home, my engineering colleagues were enjoying the new acknowledgment that they received outside the routine small parts assembly business. There were many projects initiated, but the one that had the most influence on my further training was related to the motorcar radiator.

Most folks today do not even remember driving down the highway and finding a car on the side of the road with the hood up and steam billowing into the air. This meant the radiator had become overheated, or in some cases, frozen up. One of my engineer friends worked for the Brown-Harrison Radiator Division of GM, and eventually we began to talk about the similarities between the auto radiation concept and how we could utilize it in surgery.

We had known for some time that cooling tissue reduced metabolism and, consequently, reduced the requirement for oxygen. We had been working in the dog lab on a cooling technique that would provide more time to sew in the grafts without creating damage to the vital organs, mainly the spinal cord. Putting a dog in a cold ice tub was a sloppy process; the same as it was when later applied to humans for heart surgery.

We therefore converted the auto radiation concept to a heat exchanger, where blood would flow into one end and out the other. In between tubes, cold or warm water regulated the blood temperature. The animal could be cooled and re-warmed very quickly. This is common practice in open-heart operations today as well as other clinical situations, but at that time it was very experimental.

We tested the heat exchanger built by the radiator folks and found it highly effective. However, we now knew better than to relay this information to the press, or to the dean for that matter.

4

A Cooling Experience

Over the years, medical school education has undergone dramatic changes. Nowadays, a first-year student attends a ceremony and obtains a white coat in preparation for seeing patients in the clinic and on rounds. That wasn't the case when I was going through school.

The first two years were books, examinations, and more examinations. I did not enjoy those days very much, but I continued to work in the laboratory and take call in the operating room at St. Joe's, both of which I relished greatly. At the beginning of my junior year, I was ready and eager to initiate the clinical experience. I enjoyed all the rotations, but surgery was clearly my favorite.

There was a paucity of vascular work and very little heart surgery, and as a result I became particularly intrigued with the intricacies of neurosurgery. It was probably because of the nighttime call in the operating room, where there was a preponderance of neuro cases due to trauma and intracranial bleeding.

In the lab, our experiments with the heat exchanger were working well. We were successfully cooling the animal down to protect against reduced blood flow to vital organs while replacing the arteries. I was certain that if we applied the cooling procedure to neurosurgical patients, the brain would be protected by the lowered oxygen requirement.

As a student, I was excited to tell the neurosurgical residents on rounds about the potential to rapidly cool a patient following trauma or during an operation to protect the brain. Before long the neurosurgery staff was inquiring into the "heat exchanger" idea, and soon the chief, Dr. "Eddie" Kahn, was asking me about it. We continued the experiments at St. Joe's lab, but it was not long until I received a call from Dr. Kahn's office.

"He wants you to bring your device to the operating room right away," informed his senior resident. I was so excited. I had already prepared the sterilized exchanger and was ready for action. As I approached the ER, the chief neurosurgery resident (also a good friend and mentor) rushed toward me, motioning me to go in the opposite direction.

"Ted, the old man [Dr. Kahn] wants to cool the patient who is in the ER. Take your device and run back to St. Joe's. This patient is going to die, and if you use the exchanger you will be blamed. Go now before he sees you!"

I did as recommended, and indeed the patient died. My device would have only hastened rigor mortis.

While the clinical cooling experiment was aborted for this neurosurgical patient, my work in the research laboratory continued. In fact, in 1984, more than ten years after I started the Arizona Heart Institute at St. Joseph's in Phoenix I had the perfect opportunity to prove the principal of cooling for protection during neurosurgery.

Robert Spetzler, MD, director of Barrow's Neurological Institute in Phoenix, contacted me regarding a patient who was at high risk for brain surgery. The risk was due to the potential for bleeding during repair of a large aneurysm. We discussed the concept of total body cooling with circulatory arrest (temporarily stopping the heart during the key portion of the brain procedure). We performed the operation utilizing the hypothermia approach, and the result was very satisfactory. In 1988, Dr. Spetzler published his results after using the technology in seven patients. His conclusion:

> "The perioperative morbidity and long-term results support the use of these techniques in selected patients with complex intracranial vascular lesions."

I am not certain how many of these procedures preceded ours, but it was probably one of the firsts. I know Dr. Spetzler has subsequently used this technology during similar cases.

We were nearing the end of medical school, and all my classmates were deciding on where to go for their internships and which specialty (if any) they might select for the future. My interest in blood circulation to the brain continued, and with encouragement of my friend, Dr. Ken Carrington, the chief neurosurgery resident, I made an appointment to interview with Dr. Kahn.

By now he was well aware of me, in spite of my rapid exit from the emergency case. However, the interview went well, and he offered me a position in the neurosurgical residency program. At that time there was a requirement for the resident to complete an internship, as well as one year of a general surgical residency, prior to entering the neurosurgical program. Because of my laboratory work at St. Joe's, Dr. Kahn suggested I fulfill the prerequisite requirements at St. Joe's before entering the neurosurgical residency at the University of Michigan. That seemed logical to me, and I eagerly accepted the invitation. As I was leaving his office, he said there was one other requirement: he wanted me to begin working with Dr. Elizabeth Crosby, the world famous neuroanatomist. She was located in the Kresge Research Building, right next to St. Joe's.

I could not have been happier—an appointment in neurosurgery and the opportunity to work with Dr. Crosby. It seemed like all the extra efforts beyond the ordinary school curriculum were paying off. I was accepted into the internship in 1961 and began working with Dr. Crosby whenever there was spare time.

The work with Dr. Crosby was quite different for me. While all my previous laboratory experience was done using dogs, except for a radiation experiment with rabbits, this work was on monkeys. I would sit next to Dr. Crosby, frequently referred to lovingly as "Ma Crosby," on a low stool, since she was only about four feet tall. The experiment called for stimulation of various sites in the brain, and my assignment was to follow up on the monkey twice a week, essentially performing a neurological examination to see what consequences—

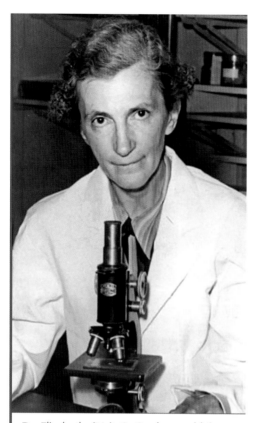

Dr. Elizabeth (Ma) C. Crosby, world famous neuroanatomist with the University of Michigan. She taught me a lot about the anatomy of the monkey's brain, but then I switched my interest to cardiovascular surgery.

positive or negative—the stimulation had created.

Not the most exciting work, but it was good preparation for the future and provided me a much better appreciation of neuroanatomy. It was actually a thrill to be working side-by-side with such a distinguished and world-respected scientist. That type of experience would be repeated many times in my future.

Working on the monkeys verified another observation that I had made from the St. Joe's emergency neuro cases and rotations with Dr. Kahn: the skull is one tough piece of bone! In order to even *get* to the brain, three circular holes were made in a triangular fashion. A special braided wire was then tunneled between the holes.

The wire, actually called a Gigli saw, was moved like flossing your teeth until a bone flap was created and removed, exposing the dura mater (the covering of the brain). This was not only a difficult procedure, but to me it seemed the antithesis of what neurosurgery should be: delicate, precise, and certainly gentle.

Since I had a research operating room at my disposal (well, it was actually under my direction at this time), I set out on a new mission to develop a saw to open the skull. We had no primates at the St. Joe's facility, so my laboratory model would have to be a canine. This turned out to be another serendipitous opportunity.

The project was far more difficult than I anticipated. First, the dog's skull seemed thicker, harder, and more difficult to cut than either the monkey or human skull. This resulted in numerous failed experiments. Basically, the sawing tool was not well designed for the dog's skull. Looking for other solutions, we purchased a saber saw at Sears and Roebuck, but this was not exactly something designed for opening the skull. A modification of the footplate next to the blade was engineered with

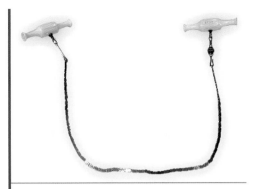

The Gigli Saw used to open the skull during brain operations.

the hope it would protect the brain, but that turned out to be hopelessly inadequate.

Time after time and dog after dog, the result was the same—poor and crude cutting of the skull and damage to the underlying tissue. I was becoming very frustrated. In fact, I began to wonder if neurosurgery was to be my career if I had to be committed to the Gigli saw.

One Saturday afternoon after more failed experiments, I had the sudden idea of trying the saw on the sternum, which is the breastbone. The canine's sternum is very narrow, and while not as hard as the skull, it's difficult to cut in a proper direction. The tools used at that time on canines, and also on clinical operating room cases, were not very sophisticated; they were more like carpenter tools. The Lebsche knife and mallet were similar to a hammer and chisel. It did work but seemed more appropriate for orthopedic procedures than for heart surgery.

I told my laboratory assistant, Jim Stanley, another student, to anesthetize a second dog and secure the paws to expose the sternum. I made the incision directly in the center of the bone and placed the footplate at the lower end of the sternum.

The power was turned on, and like magic the saw made a perfect separation of the bone. No bleeding, no injury to the pericardium, the covering of the heart, or the heart itself.

It was fantastic, so we anesthetized another animal with similar perfect results. One more trial resulted in one more perfect performance of the saw. Three for three was enough for me. I picked up the phone and called my friend Joe Morris.

"Joe, you have to come to the lab after church in the morning. I have something unbelievable to show you." He came over the next day and we repeated the experiment two more times. His parting words were, "Ted, I'll give you a call," but the call came sooner than I expected. He told me he had a substernal goiter to remove on an elderly lady Monday morning. Did I think the saw would work? I was sure the saw would work.

At 11 a.m. on Monday, I proved the potential for the Sternal Saw with perfect exposure of the tumor and no complications. On Thursday, Dr. Morris had an adult ASD (hole in the heart) where I used the saw, again observing a perfect result.

Telling this story and the history that follows almost blurs the ink on the paper. Can you imagine any such experience happening today? There's no way, not with the Food and Drug Administration's (FDA) endless regulatory hurdles and countless obstacles to overcome. Are we better off now than in the 1950s? A discussion for another chapter, but the Sternal Saw certainly made history.

An interesting note here: eventually, my laboratory assistant Jim Stanley became Professor of Surgery at the University of Michigan and head of the Department of Vascular Surgery. He was also instrumental in creating the Cardiovascular Research Center there. Many years later, he graciously invited me to be a member of their advisory board.

The Lebsche knife used to split the breastbone in open-heart procedures seen here with the surgical mallet.

5

The Music Stand

I f the central themes of this story are not patently clear by now, then I have failed to accomplish my mission. There are three themes woven throughout this book which are the essential ingredients in my life's work: medicine, music, and sports. The "music stand" exemplifies a portion of these themes.

There was no question that my senior year of medical school was a high point in my education. For the first time, I began to understand what it would feel like to be a real doctor.

While many of my rotations were on surgical services by my choice, there was one exceptional experience when I was chosen for a unique program in the general surgery department. About a dozen of the senior students were selected to rotate on the professor's service, not as students, but in a "special" elevated position, like a junior intern working directly with the first-year surgical residents. I'm not sure if it had been tried before or if it was an experiment, but for me it was an unbelievable opportunity—working with the patients, writing orders, observing and assisting in the operating room, and most important, being around some of the most famous surgeons of that time.

Me, a senior medical student, standing side-by-side at the operating table with the most respected of the profession? I didn't ever want to leave the hospital, choosing instead to work around the clock, something that would be strongly forbidden today. Surrounded by my heroes, it was like the beginning of my dreams coming true.

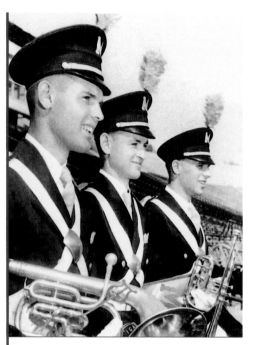
In the lineup for the Michigan Marching Band.

Then suddenly, the bubble burst in a most unanticipated way. Maybe it was an example of reverse serendipity, where an event unexpectedly spins in a negative direction.

The conductor of Michigan Marching Band (1935–1971), Professor William D. Revelli, was another one of my heroes, but in quite a different specialty. He set the standard of excellence for the Michigan Marching Band, and perfection was prevalent in every note of the musical performances, every eight steps per ten yards on the football field. The Michigan Marching Band won international acclaim for its musical precision under his leadership. Once again, sports and music are joined. Nobody can capture that synapse better than the story, "Revelli Teaches 'The Victors' to the Football Team":

When Bo Schembechler was hired as Michigan's football coach in 1969, Revelli was the first person to visit him when he arrived at his new office: "I'm in my office, and the first visitor that I get, the absolute first visitor is William D. Revelli." Revelli sat down and said, "I want you to know that I coach my band exactly the same way you coach your football team. We'll have discipline, and we'll do it the way it's supposed to be done!" Revelli added, "Anything you need from me or the band, all you need to do is ask."

When the freshmen arrived in the fall of 1969, Schembechler asked Revelli to teach them how to sing "The Victors." Schembechler said, "He didn't just teach them 'The Victors.' He taught them Michigan tradition!" Schembechler gathered the freshmen at Yost Field House, and Revelli entered in full uniform—described by Schembechler as "a lean, short, and distinguished-looking older gentleman—a band director right out of central casting."

Revelli rose to the podium, tapped his baton, looked right into their eyes and said, "John Philip Sousa called this the greatest fight song ever written. And you will sing it with respect!" Revelli brought out a

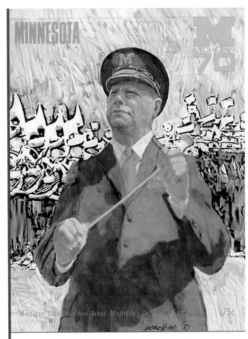

Revelli on the Michigan Stadium game program, October 1970.

pitch pipe and began the instructions. "You sing from down in here, in your diaphragm. You bring it up from down here with feeling." Then he blew the starting note on his pitch pipe. The players started, "Hail to the Victors, valiant—" Revelli interrupted, "No, No, No! That's terrible! There's no enthusiasm, you didn't sing with enthusiasm!" They started again, and Revelli interrupted again. "No, no, no! We're gonna get this right if I'm here all night!"

Schembechler thought so much of Revelli's performance that he invited him back every year to teach the freshmen what Michigan tradition was about. Schembechler recalled, "He was absolutely great, and the freshmen absolutely loved it. And let me tell you, every one of those freshmen came out of that session with Revelli knowing 'The Victors.' They knew the words, they knew how to sing it, and they knew how to emphasize the right spots. They flat out knew how to do it. And it was only because he came over there with the idea that those

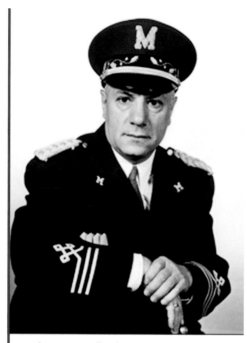

Professor Revelli, director of the Michigan Marching Band.

guys were going to come out of that meeting room knowing how to sing this fight song the right way or else! And they did. That was Bill Revelli."

The admiration between Revelli and Schembechler was mutual. In a 1970 interview, Revelli compared himself and his training methods to those of Schembechler. "Bo and I speak the same language. Psychologically, our practices are the same. Both the team and the band have to perfect their fundamentals before they can do anything else. And both need proper warmups to stay in shape in the off-season. We'll spend forty-five minutes on calisthenics of the embouchure (perfecting the position of the lips on the mouthpiece of an instrument). I had one boy come back who hadn't practiced all summer. His lips were about six months behind everyone else's."

Revelli acknowledged the performance of the Ohio script and the dotting of the "i" to the Ohio State Marching Band on the football field. Beyond that it was an all out battle of the bands, and at times even more important than the numbers on the scoreboard. Yes, Revelli was the initiator of synchronized music and movement on the football field. He was also the first to use an announcer, and you could hear it ten times every fall: "Band, take the field!"

Frequently, the fans cheered louder for the band than for the football team. During one half time we played and danced to the then hit song, "Rock Around The Clock."

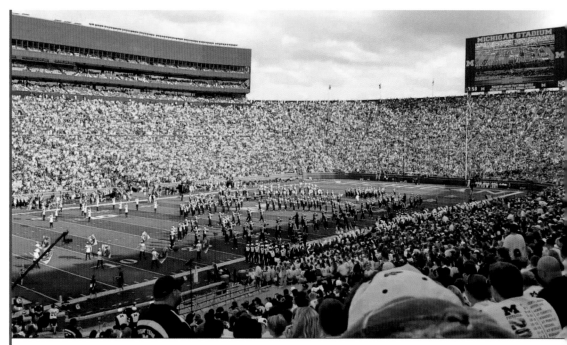

Michigan Marching Band at center stage of the Big House in the modern era.

As the football team came out of the tunnel to reenter, the referees had to form a barrier because the band was still at the center of the field. The fans from end zone to end zone were shouting and cheering for a repeat of the hit song! Revelli stood his ground and motioned to the drum major to give four short bursts on his whistle indicating the band should replay "Rock Around The Clock." The fans went wild! The football team stood on the sidelines as if saluting their marching band. At the end of the day, they were both victorious, two teams representing the great University of Michigan and all its traditions since 1817.

We used the music stands for inside rehearsal or music lyres on our horns during the early part of the week. By mid-week, usually Wednesdays, we took to the practice field for live marching practice. Our schedule was similar to that of the football team's, except when it rained, they stayed inside.

By Friday it was all by memory, and the music books were left on the sidelines. However, if the sound of the music was less than Professor Revelli's expectations he would demand that every player report to his office for a personal performance of the half time show. The quality of the Saturday performance under Professor Revelli's direction revealed his obsession with perfection, and the absence of the music stands and lyre crutches were the signal that his team had come to play.

Fast-forward three years, after I had experienced the thrill of performing in the "Big House" (it was not yet called that in those days) during football games with the Michigan Marching Band. Now I was on a special service of the surgical professors. I stayed up all night studying surgical books and drawings about the case the professors were going to perform the next morning. It was scheduled as a brachial artery repair, a vascular case, the area I had been working on for several years at St. Joe's lab with Dr. Crook. I had no idea what to expect. While the professors were extremely accessible to this special group of senior students, especially rotating between them and the residents, there still was the natural distance between the two.

I was the first person in the operating room after the nurses. I had the patient's record memorized, much like the music for the Saturday football performance. I placed x-rays on the view box and then talked to the anesthesia resident and the nurses. There was a high level of tension. It was not only because of the uncertainties of the procedure, but the fact that this was the first vascular procedure performed by the new head of the Department of General Surgery at the University. The world-famous Professor Frederic A. Coller had retired and was being replaced by C. Gardner Child III from Tufts University in Boston. Dr. DeWeis, another professor, was scheduled as the first assistant. My name did not appear on the operating schedule.

The patient was anesthetized. The left arm was draped out to the side on a special arm support and prepped for the procedure. The room was becoming more crowded. Dr. DeWeis came in after scrubbing, looked at the x-rays, and then left the room.

Without announcement or fanfare, Professor Child walked through the double doors, an anatomy textbook in his left hand and a music stand in his right. With some pomp and circumstance, he adjusted the music stand, opened the anatomy book to a page previously marked, and adjusted it in a position where he would have an unobstructed view of the anatomic drawing as he stood next to the outstretched, supported arm. Dr. DeWeis reappeared almost simultaneously, also without announcement.

I had already positioned myself as close as possible to the operative side, making sure to stand behind the senior resident. As this operative saga continued to unfold, I could not believe what I was witnessing.

The surgeons were mumbling about something, and one asked the circulating nurse to turn the page of the surgical anatomy book on the music stand. I peeked over the senior resident's shoulder for a better view. Were my eyes deceiving me? I had studied most of the night in the same way I practiced before band performances. These two famous surgeons were using anatomic drawings in the operating room, supported by a music stand?

Professor Revelli had every note of every piece of music embedded into his brain when the band took the field. No music stands. Every note played perfectly.

I left the operating room that morning with profoundly mixed emotions. On one hand, my expectations and images of the master surgeons were somewhat shattered. On the other hand, the respect for the professionalism and perfection of my music professor was reinforced.

To be sure, that day I committed never to use a music stand.

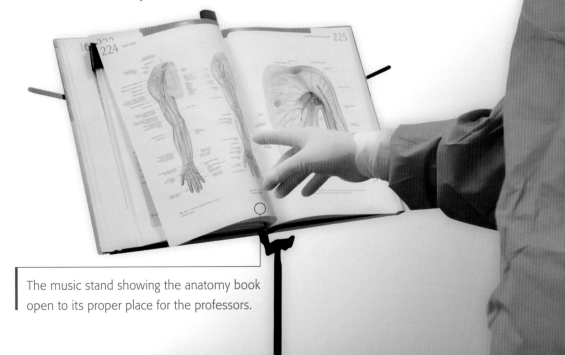

The music stand showing the anatomy book
open to its proper place for the professors.

6

The Game Changer

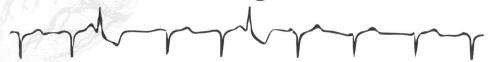

The success of the Sternal Saw at the University was an important element of the beginning of my relationship with bioengineering.

In his true neighborly fashion, Dick Sarns provided me with an invaluable sounding board for the practicality of new ideas. At the same time, I was becoming more convinced that perhaps neurosurgery was not the best long-term career choice. It may seem strange that the ease to split the sternum and the inability to open the skull would be a game changer for me in selecting a surgical career path. In truth, there were several other factors.

Our medical fraternity sponsored visiting professors who came to speak on their area of expertise. On one specific occasion, I listened to Dr. Robert Gross from Boston Children's Hospital describe his procedure to correct a congenital arterial defect, and also the experimentation with the heart/lung machine. It was so fascinating and right in sync with what we had been doing in the dog lab.

Suddenly it all came together: I was not destined to become a neurosurgeon. Instead of chasing the pithed primates for neurological examination, I was to be petting the barrel-chested Boxer that awakened from an operation to test a new heart/lung machine.

Once I realized this, I knew what must be done. First I had to visit Dr. Kahn with an explanation for the change in my future plans. Then I needed to obtain an all-important interview with Professor Cameron Haight, the head of thoracic surgery at the University of Michigan, because a thoracic residency was the pathway to becoming a cardiovascular surgeon. In addition, I wanted to start the Sarns Company with my neighbor Dick to continue our advancements, and finally my general surgery residency at St. Joe's would have to be expanded from one to four years before I could even enter a thoracic residency program. Now I was committed to seven more years of training—at a minimum.

I made my decision in 1961. One afternoon, I was rotating on the various surgical services for my internship at St. Joe's when one of the nurses flagged me down. "Do you know who the patient is in Room 402? It's Professor Henry Ranson's patient, scheduled for a breast biopsy in the morning," she said excitedly. "She is Dr. Emerik Szilagyi's wife. He is the famous vascular surgeon from Henry Ford Hospital in Detroit." She did not need to tell me about him; I had already become acquainted with his reputation. This particular nurse knew of my interest in vascular surgery and had in fact helped in the lab. It was at that moment another serendipitous event came into play.

The nurse suggested that I go in and introduce myself to Mrs. Szilagyi. I did just that, and explained to Mrs. Szilagyi that I would like to spend some time studying with her husband at Henry Ford's, only forty miles or so from Ann Arbor. She suggested I write a letter directly to him. So I wrote a nice introductory letter... and received a terrible response:

"Like who do you think you are? We have a formal residency program here. We have no intentions of taking people from the outside. Out of the question!"

That is just a mild flavor of the epistle. Some may say he was just in a bad mood, but later I learned he was a tough Hungarian.

At the time there were really only a few vascular surgeons recognized for outstanding work. One was Michael DeBakey in Houston, while another was Szilagyi, who had originally rejected my letter, but I wasn't going to accept a "no" without even a face-to-face interview. I called his secretary, introduced myself, and explained I had received a rejection letter. She was already aware of that, of course, and did sound at least a little sympathetic.

"Could I make an appointment to meet with him?" I asked.

"Doubt that it can be arranged. He is very busy," she responded.

After begging, several calls and more letters (and getting to know her in the process), I received the interview appointment. By the time I entered Dr. Szilagyi's office that Saturday morning, there wasn't anything on paper he had written that I had not read. I was prepared like I was taking the surgical examinations. At first, he was rather abrupt and grumpy as expected, but after the proper answer to some tough questions, I could see some sunlight through the clouds. He laid out the conditions.

First, I would have to perform as one of their residents: six months, nighttime call, rounds, and operative assisting. Second, I had to learn and participate in the angiographic studies. How could I ask for more? It was the opportunity of a lifetime, except for the disruption of having to leave Gloria and our two children in Ann Arbor to drive back and forth when I was not on call. But after six months, when I returned to St. Joe's and the University, I knew more about vascular surgery and angiography than anyone on the campus and beyond.

In those early years, all angiograms were done by direct-needle puncture into the aorta, followed by injection of dye. On November 22 in 1963, I was in the x-ray room having just performed an angiogram. A nurse appeared at the door announcing that President Kennedy had been killed. That news made the angiogram results seem inconsequential.

The fourth year of residency back at St. Joe's was the most exciting, because as the senior resident I had my choice of which operations and surgeons I wanted to work with. All of the attending surgeons were very good, but my favorite was Dr. Darrell Campbell. He had gone through the U of M general surgery program under the direction of Dr. Coller. Many said he was one of Dr. Coller's all-time favorites. He was technically superb, but more important (at least to me), he had an interest in vascular surgery.

When I returned from Henry Ford and Dr. Szilagyi's program, Dr. Campbell really took me under his wing. He was my first assistant on every case, particularly the vascular cases. He was like a father, advising me in all aspects of surgery and even business. On the latter he made a mistake. Dr. Campbell advised me against being involved in a commercial enterprise. Doctors did not do that. Indeed, it was early in the game, but more on that later.

The Sarns Company was progressing very well, on track to become a leading manufacturer of heart-lung equipment. I spent considerable time working with the company on new products, but the Sternal Saw was a market leader, particularly after I published an article extolling its virtues.

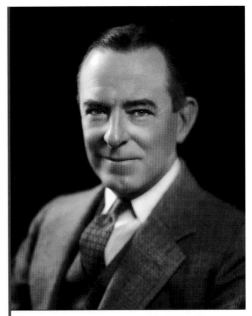

Frederick A. Coller, MD, co-founder of the American College of Surgeons.

It was clear that the unorthodox rotation with Dr. Szilagyi had propelled my technical skills to a new level, but at the same time it presented confusion for my future training and career. The specialty of cardiovascular surgery was ill defined, and it was just getting its start at the university.

The vascular surgery program at Henry Ford only covered the abdomen to the toes, while Dr. Haight's program at Michigan was strongly oriented toward surgery for lung and esophageal problems. On the other hand, Baylor College of Medicine in Houston, where Dr. DeBakey was chairman, emphasized both adult cardiac and vascular surgery. Additionally, pediatric surgery was emphasized under Dr. Denton Cooley's tutelage. Houston was where the most advanced arterial procedures were performed by an outstanding group of surgeons.

I explored my opportunities, looking at which residency programs would be available after I finished my chief surgical year. That's when I came across a surgical atlas published by Dr. DeBakey.

It was devoted exclusively to vascular repair of obstructions and aneurysms in both the chest and abdomen. It was more than 250 pages, black and white, with

Reprinted from SURGERY, St. Louis
Vol. 53, No. 5, Pages 637-638, May, 1963. (Printed in the U. S. A.)
(Copyright © 1963 by The C. V. Mosby Company)

Sternal saw—new instrument for splitting the sternum

EDWARD B. DIETHRICH, M.D.
JOE D. MORRIS, M.D.

ANN ARBOR, MICH.

From the Department of Surgery, St. Joseph Mercy Hospital

Midline sternotomy is the approach of choice in the correction of many congenital and acquired defects of the heart and great vessels. While the sternum may be divided manually with knives, chisels, shears, and various power instruments, no completely satisfactory instrument has been reported to date. This report describes a new instrument designed expressly for splitting the sternum during approach to the anterior mediastinum. It has been used clinically with gratifying results in over 250 operations.

The sternal saw* (Fig. 1) is a compact unit weighing one pound. It is constructed entirely of noncorrosive materials. The pistol type design permits it to be held in one hand and allows maximum maneuverability.

Power is supplied by a ⅛ h.p. Foredom motor or by a conventional Stryker motor. The reciprocating blade is driven by a double eccentric counter-weighted cam from the power source. The blade reciprocates 5,000 strokes per minute with a stroke length of 5 mm. Because of this rapid, short movement, the blade cuts the solid sternum but will not harm the soft tissues.

A snub-nosed footpiece adds stability to the blade in addition to pushing aside underlying structures. The serrated blade does not clog with bony material and the cut is smooth and relatively bloodless.

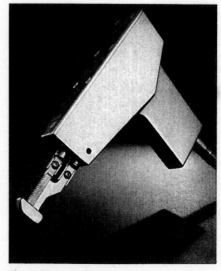

Fig. 1. The sternal saw.

The saw, blade, and flexible cable are completely autoclavable. The sterile flexible cable is passed from the operating table to the motor prior to use. All cable connections are the quick disconnect type for rapid assembly and disassembly. The unit requires no lubrication. Removing a single screw permits separating the blade from the saw for cleaning. The entire unit is washed under running water.

Supported in part by the Edgar A. Kahn Neurosurgical Fund.
Received for publication July 30, 1962.
*Built by Sarns, Inc., Ann Arbor, Mich.

pen and ink drawings. No text had been printed like it before. It became my "Bible." The map of what I wanted for the future.

I would become a cardiovascular surgeon, taking care of and operating on patients with heart and blood vessel disease. I would be part of the embryonic specialty, where I could combine my interest of biomedical engineering with advanced skills and techniques in the operating room.

I searched for other "Bibles" that I could use throughout the East Coast, West Coast, and even Europe. There were many training programs, but

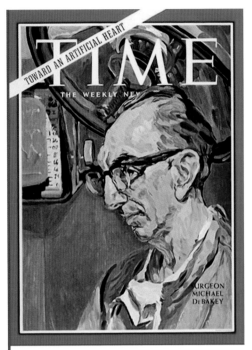

Dr. Michael DeBakey on the cover of *TIME* magazine the same year I arrived at Baylor to begin my training in his department.

none that I felt matched what I envisioned in Houston. Was I being unrealistic? I had turned down a position in the university neurosurgery department under Dr. Kahn, and Dr. Haight had already "reserved" a thoracic residency spot for me next July. Most young surgical trainees would have been ecstatic with those potentials.

The same unrest that I had witnessed with the Dr. Szilagyi position was spawned all over again. So I completed the application for the cardiothoracic residency at Baylor College of Medicine where Dr. Michael DeBakey was the department professor and chairman. I felt like I was writing to Moses, the famous Biblical author.

To the contrary of my Henry Ford experience, a response was quickly received and a date to meet Dr. DeBakey was set. The first person to know was Gloria, and the second was Dr. Campbell, as I was seeking his advice throughout this process.

Gloria and I left for Houston with an intermediary stop in St. Louis. I got off the plane to pick up some reading material, and there on the rack was the current

May issue of *TIME* magazine 1965. On the cover was Dr. Michael E. DeBakey announcing the initiation of Medicare.

There I was, going to interview for a residency program with not only one of the most famous surgeons in the world, but also one who was about to shape the future of our health care system. However, as I am writing this today, it is not certain to me if we have made a great deal of progress on that front.

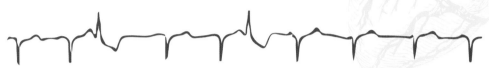

The Non-Interview

We checked into the Shamrock Hotel near Methodist Hospital. First thing the next morning I walked to the hospital in my coat and tie. It was my first introduction to the Houston humidity, and the anticipation of meeting Dr. DeBakey only added to the uncomfortable feeling.

I found Dr. DeBakey's office rather easily and was greeted by his secretary Polly. Soon his administrative assistant Jerry Maley entered the room. I had hardly said hello before he explained that Dr. DeBakey was operating on a Greek Air Force captain, and he wanted me to go upstairs to the dome over the operating room.

"He will meet you after he's finished with the procedure," Jerry added.

As I went up the back steps to the dome, I felt like it was the most exciting day of my life. I was going to see Dr. DeBakey operate to repair an aortic arch aneurysm, the very type of procedures we were doing in our lab and I had reviewed in his atlas.

Up in the dome, my face was pressed against the glass. I watched every move of my (hopefully) future mentor. Suddenly, he left the operating room. I flew down the back stairs—actually almost tripping on them—knowing he would be looking for me. But he was nowhere to be seen. Maybe he just needed a bathroom break. Back up the stairs I flew to the dome. This went on all day, up and down, but I didn't mind. I was watching the greatest surgeon in the world.

Later in the afternoon I could see the procedure was concluding. I sprinted down the stairs and ran right into Jerry. I explained I had not seen Dr. DeBakey yet, and he replied that the doctor was in the intensive care unit, but wanted to see me first thing in the morning.

The next day was a repeat of the first. Up and down the steps I went, watching the operations. Still, there was no contact with Dr. DeBakey. Late in the afternoon I saw Jerry and explained that, due to my call schedule, I had to leave for Ann Arbor early in the morning.

"He will definitely see you tomorrow, don't worry," he reassured.

Early the next morning we packed and went to the hospital. As I looked down the corridor I saw Dr. DeBakey and Jerry headed my way. I was sure they were looking for me. I waved my arms so they couldn't miss me.

As they approached, Jerry Maley made the introductions. "Dr. DeBakey, this is Dr. Diethrich from the University of Michigan. He is here for a residency interview." Dr. DeBakey looked up, said, "Nice to see you," and walked on. No handshakes, no smile, and most important, no interview.

The flight back to Detroit was a long one—not so much in actual flight time, but exhaustion over my situation. As my mind reeled, I reviewed my situation: I had given up a prestigious neurosurgical residency position with Dr. Kahn and perhaps provoked Dr. Haight by not immediately accepting the position in the thoracic surgery program at the University of Michigan. Before going to Houston for the intended interview, Dr. Haight had called me to his office. He was leaving for a trip to Italy, and unless I accepted the position within the week, he was going to offer it to one of the other dozen or so candidates.

Was I on the precipice of missing my chance to explore my new life ambition in cardiovascular surgery?

By the time I returned to St. Joe's the next morning, I had a plan. I was going to meet with Dr. Campbell and get his advice. After all, he was my best friend and surgical mentor, as well as one of the most respected surgeons on the staff. He had that close relationship with Dr. Coller, whose office was right next to his. Dr. Coller was a co-founder of the American College of Surgeons, and as such, was one of the most important surgeons of the time.

Dr. Campbell appreciated that I was in a pickle. A wrong move could prove fatal to my career.

"Ted, go to Dr. Coller's office next door and ask for his advice. He is one of the senior surgeons in the United States, if not in the world. He also likes you and knows of your laboratory work downstairs." Indeed, he had visited me on several occasions when we were working on new devices.

I didn't hesitate. Time was running out and I needed to execute the three-minute drill. Fortunately, Dr. Coller was sitting at his desk when I knocked on the door. He invited me in with his usual hoarse voice, suffering from asthma and COPD.

"What can I do for you, Ted?"

I explained my predicament. He was quiet for a moment or two and then clearly said, "Do nothing, just wait for now."

What are the longest days of the week when you are waiting for the answer to a critical question? They are all the same, filled with some uncontrolled angst. On Thursday and Friday, I could hardly concentrate on my work.

On Saturday morning, Dr. Campbell and I did the usual rounds. We were about halfway through seeing the patients when I had an overhead page for a phone message. No cell phones in those days. I answered, and it was Gloria.

"Ted, you have a letter from the Department of Surgery, Baylor College of Medicine, Dr. Michael E. DeBakey."

"What does it say?" I asked.

"I don't know, I didn't open it." She was often the last person to open her presents on Christmas morning. Such patience—maybe that's why she tolerated me all these years!

"Open it!" I nearly yelled.

Gloria cleared her throat and began reading the letter.

"Dear Dr. Diethrich, you have been accepted into the thoracic and cardiovascular residency program at Baylor College of Medicine. Your appointment will begin July 1, 1965. Sincerely, Michael E. DeBakey, MD, Chairman."

I was in a "drop dead" state. I spoke confidentially with Dr. Campbell and asked him to excuse me from rounds. I had to see Dr. Coller. I called his home and asked Mrs. Coller if I could come over.

"It's not a good time, he feels poorly and is coughing," she explained.

"I will only be two minutes," I pleaded.

She finally relented, and I was at the front door in 10 minutes. She greeted me and escorted me to the second floor bedroom.

Mrs. Coller was right. He was not feeling well; you could tell from the way he looked. I approached his bed and apologized for the interruption.

"I'll only take a moment of your time, but I wanted you to know that I received an acceptance letter to Dr. DeBakey's program." He was very quiet. Adjusting his head on the pillows, he cleared his throat and looked directly into my eyes.

"Today, my boy, you learned a great lesson. It is not what you know—but who!" I did not ask and he did not tell. Had a phone call been made? At this point it did not matter. A great lesson had been learned. That was one of so many lessons I learned at Michigan.

The opportunities in research, instrument development, and the gaining of surgical skills certainly laid the foundation for the next steps in my life. Dr. Coller, in my interview with him regarding Dr. DeBakey, had taught me a lesson but so much of what I learned really was by personal experiences. On nearly the last day at St. Joseph's Hospital and the completion of my year as senior resident I was called urgently to see Dr. Coller in a hospital room. When I arrived, Dr. Campbell was already present. The urgency related to the fact that the Grand Professor had an "acute abdomen" meaning that something very serious was wrong and it would require an emergency operation. I sprang into action and notified the operating room and the anesthesiologist Dr. Ed Krigbaum, one of the best I have ever known. Within an hour the professor was transferred to the operating room and the OR team assembled. As senior resident I went over all the details of the laboratory work, x-rays, and the operative plan.

There was no definitive diagnosis but there was high suspicion that we were dealing with a HOT gallbladder that required immediate removal. I was first to scrub in after the instrument nurse. I applied the sterile drapes which were positioned perfectly. (See Chapter 8: "Entering the World of Michael Ellis DeBakey" for a later account of draping a patient. Quite a different story then.)

Dr. Krigbaum acknowledged that Dr. Coller was hemodynamically stable and the operation could begin. I was standing at attention with my hands on the operating table when I suddenly looked around the room. There, peering back at me were four professors of surgery including Dr. Coller's partner. They all stood at a similar attention position that I had assumed. There was no conversation, maybe some whispering that I could not hear. After several minutes that seemed like hours, the reality of the situation dawned on me. These were some of the finest surgeons in the world. All students of Dr. Coller but not one of them was scrubbed to begin the operation. I knew each of them very well and any one of them could have performed the procedure as well as the next. The problem, this was Dr. Coller, The Chief, The Professor, and the founder of the American College of Surgeons. Who was to take the lead?

Ed Krigbaum bent his head over the drape at the head of the table. "Ted, I suggest you make the incision so we can get on with the procedure." I looked around the room again as the scrub nurse put the scalpel in my hand. I glanced up at Dr. Campbell who was suddenly giving me a positive nod. The operation had begun and without fanfare three of Dr. Coller's most famous professors were standing next to me, each ready to remove the ugly, inflamed gallbladder. I assumed the usual location of the senior resident next to the professor who finally accepted his customary position at the head of the operating table.

Dr. Coller recovered without any serious complications in spite of his chronic lung disease. It was an exciting incident for me, and little did I know that within a year I would be faced with another critical decision about initiating an operation, but this time not surrounded by professors but rather encouraged by fellow trainees in the dome above the operating room next to where Dr. DeBakey was performing a cardiac procedure. (See Chapter 8: "Entering the World of Michael Ellis DeBakey.")

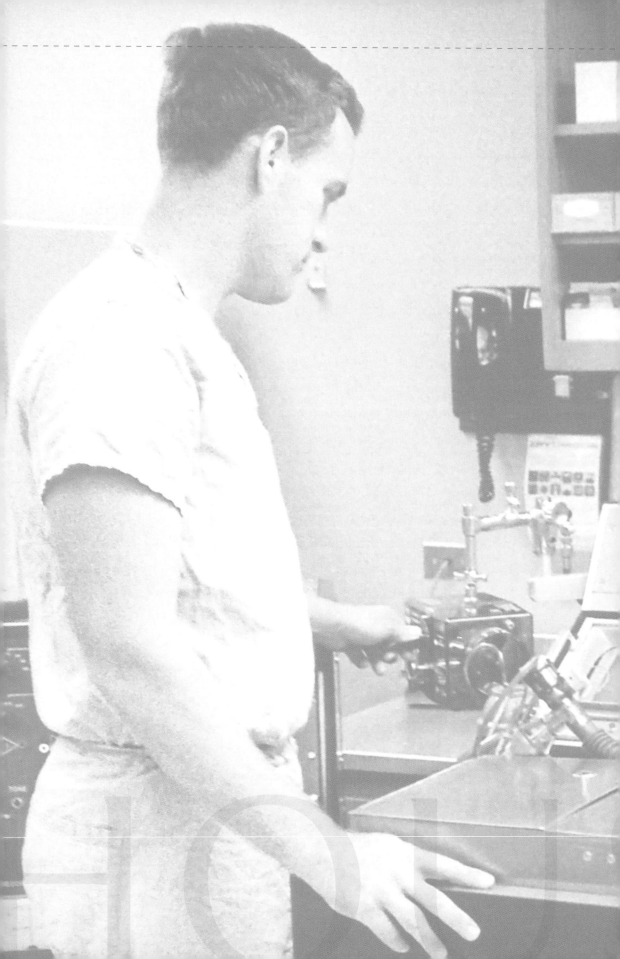

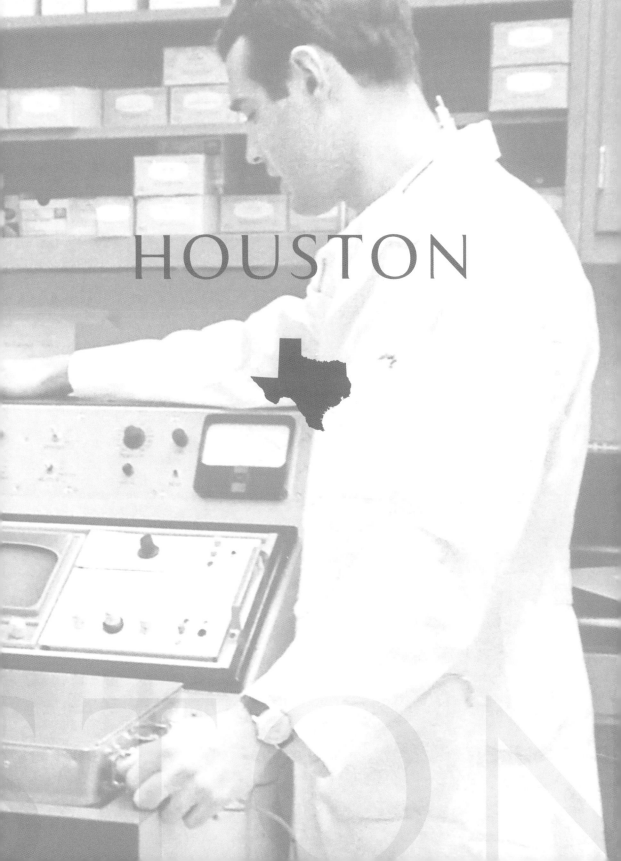

HOUSTON

8
Entering the World of
Dr. Michael Ellis DeBakey

At the Baylor Thoracic and Cardiovascular program, the board required a two-year residency. There were four residents at the first year level and four at the second. During my first year I was to rotate on Dr. Cooley's service at St. Luke's and Texas Children's Hospitals. They were actually connected by a tunnel to the Methodist Hospital, which was Dr. DeBakey's main facility.

The other rotations were with the VA program for chest and esophageal surgery, and the Ben Taub Hospital, a charity facility with a very active emergency department. The Methodist Hospital with Dr. DeBakey was the fourth component of my first-year schedule.

How fortunate it was that my first rotation assignment was with Dr. Cooley. I had met him at the American College of Surgeons Congress in San Francisco the same year I had the scientific exhibit on the shunt clamp project.

As I entered the operating area of St. Luke's Hospital, the first person I saw was Dr. Cooley. I introduced myself as his first-year resident for the initial rotation, and he began sizing me up, head to waist. Unbelievably, he soon handed me my scrub pants and shirt.

Dr. Denton Cooley, the consummate teacher and a good friend.

Can you imagine, the head surgeon picking out the scrubs for the first-year resident? That brief experience taught me a great deal about his character. He was not only a world-class surgeon, he was a world-class gentleman.

Already I had encountered outstanding professors and teachers along the way, and I was developing a mental catalog of their traits. I couldn't help but think to myself: Could I emulate the qualities of these stars in my future practice?

The next morning I was the first assistant on a pediatric vascular case and on my third day, he said, "Ted, yesterday you saw one, today you did one, and tomorrow you'll teach one." See one, do one, teach one was his motto.

After a few days on this rotation, I wrote to one of my former resident colleagues back in Michigan:

"I thought we in Ann Arbor were really good, but we are not even on the same planet as these Houston surgeons. No wonder surgeons from every country around the world are coming here to observe and learn. I definitely made the correct choice and I am so lucky."

My second rotation was at the Veteran's Hospital, where the focus was mostly on lung surgery and treatment of tuberculosis. There was no cardiovascular, so I had time to begin some laboratory work over at the school.

By mid-December I was scheduled to go to the Ben Taub County Hospital for the third rotation, when I received a call from a first-year colleague, Charley McCollum. We had only recently met, and he had gone through the Baylor general surgery program and was currently on Dr. DeBakey's service at my level. McCollum said it was critical that I talk to him that afternoon, and while he did not volunteer an explanation, he certainly sounded upset. We arranged a meeting at the school office.

"Ted, you have to do me a great favor. The old man [Dr. DeBakey] is going to fire me any minute now. A patient died and he is blaming me," McCollum explained. "It wasn't my fault, but that doesn't really matter. He wants me out of here right now."

I responded with sympathy because I had heard that Dr. DeBakey was notorious for suddenly discharging trainees. But how could I help?

"Your next rotation is County, so how about I go there starting the weekend after Christmas and you replace me at Methodist," he suggested, answering my question. "If I get out of his sight, he may forget this issue and let me complete my residency."

What Charley was suggesting seemed impossible to me. I hardly knew where Methodist Hospital was, let alone any of its internal workings. Charley had been at Baylor for years and was well acquainted with the doctors and nurses and all the intricacies of the institution. He had also worked with Dr. DeBakey on several previous rotations. Charley didn't explain the situation any further, but it sounded like I could be stepping into a potential path of termination myself, the very one he was trying to avoid. However, he seemed so desperate that I could not refuse. There would be only a few days before the next rotations started on January 1. I could easily leave the VA rotation early, so I did. Then began the camp out.

On Dr. DeBakey's rotation, the first-year cardiovascular resident "ran" his service. This meant that he or she was responsible for all activity on the service. It was not uncommon to have fifty to sixty patients in various stages of preoperative, operative, and postoperative care. That resident reported directly to Dr. DeBakey, twenty-four hours a day. There were interns, junior, or second-year cardiovascular residents, but the buck stopped with that first-year cardiovascular resident.

Due to the holidays, things were rather calm at the Methodist Hospital. It gave me a chance to talk to Polly, Dr. DeBakey's secretary, and get her views on a "survival kit." Clearly she was the most important daily spoke in the DeBakey wheel. I did not leave the hospital at all. In fact, Gloria and the kids came to the hospital to eat with me in the cafeteria. I introduced myself to every nurse and doctor, explaining my new role at the hospital.

Almost universally, I was greeted with raised eyebrows, rolling eyes, and a very weak "best of luck" greeting. Not at all different than what I expected after speaking with Polly. She had seen many residents come and go, and it appeared I was the first one taken in the thoracic program who had not done some general surgery training at Baylor. I was an outsider of sorts, not unlike my experience with

Dr. Szilagy, but that worked out fine. This might also, and if hard work was the key, I would be okay.

On my first official morning I was prepared to meet him. There was not a single item about any patient that I could not recite with a snap. Polly had typed the "rounds list" several times because I wanted it to be perfect. That was key, because the patient's location, status, and plan were listed, and I was to direct Dr. DeBakey to each room and give him a verbal report. It was a routine repeated every afternoon.

His office was off a hallway from the elevator. There was the secretary's area and a smaller office complete with a chart working section and x-ray view box where the resident sat. Dr. DeBakey's office door, always locked, was directly adjacent to the resident's seat. That may seem inconsequential, but not so.

I heard him coming down the hallway, and as he turned toward his office door and put the key in the lock, he looked down at me. I started to speak but he opened the door, disappeared inside, and slammed it shut. When the door opened again, I quickly stood up.

"Dr. DeBakey. I'm Dr. Diethrich, your resident for this rotation. I have the rounds prepared," I said in a clear voice. Together we went over the list, looked at the x-rays, and left the office to see the patients. I made sure that I was always a half-step ahead with list in hand.

"Dr. DeBakey, this is Mr. Smith. He is scheduled for an abdominal aneurysm repair in the a.m." He would go in, examine the patient, and explain the plan. Then it was on to the next room with some questions about blood count, kidney function, and so forth, but I had every answer.

Rounds completed, he went off to the operating room, and I reported back to Polly with a sigh of relief. It seemingly had gone perfect, but then again, he couldn't ask me a question I didn't know. I had ensured I was prepared.

The first three or four days continued well. He didn't say anything negative to me; all was quiet. It was going to be everything I had hoped it would be. I was in the presence of the master. Little did I know I was about to enter the gates of hell, and it was to be the worst experience of my whole life.

In early January, somebody said, maybe it was Polly, "Ted, you need to start scrubbing, you can't spend all the time just taking care of the patients." So I scrubbed the next day as a second assistant on a heart case. My routine became scrubbing in the morning, rounds in the afternoons.

In the third week of my rotation, I was again the second assistant on a mitral valve replacement. Suddenly DeBakey stopped the operation and looked at me.

"Well, Dr. Diethrich, don't you know how to hold the retractor? How can I do this operation if you can't give me exposure?" he demanded.

I could never seem to make it through a case with him—I'd make the incision wrong, I couldn't hold a retractor, or I was standing in his light. Everything was wrong. He'd say, "Why can't you do this for me, doctor, why, why, WHY?" or "Don't you want to help me, doctor? This doctor doesn't want to help me!" he would shout to the operating room staff. We'd start a case and about ten minutes into it, he'd stop, throw up his hands and say, "Ted, would you get Dr. Garrett?" Somebody would go get Dr. Garrett, and Dr. DeBakey would banish me to a corner. "You just stand over there, doctor."

It got to the point where I lost all my confidence. He could shatter you, absolutely shatter you. He would say to the whole operating room, "It must be intentional—nobody could operate like this unless it was intentional." But I never answered back to him. I never raised my voice because that provoked him the most.

This went on day after day after day, until one afternoon he laid down the instruments and said, "All right, doctor, all right. This is it. This is it! You operate, and I'm going to assist you. Here, you take these forceps, and you take this needle, and you take this suture, and you sew up the artery."

I started in. It lasted about thirty seconds before he grabbed everything back from me.

It is difficult to express how demeaning this experience was for me. It got so bad that he wouldn't even let me drape the patient, something I had been doing for years. It was as routine as taking a temperature. Draping a patient for an operation is fundamental in the earliest days of surgical training. I hold the all-time record for draping a patient!

Then it happened. One Saturday morning Dr. DeBakey was going to perform a carotid endarterectomy. I scrubbed and draped as we always did. He came in to the room, took one look at the drapes, and tore them off. After he stormed out, I asked the nurse what I had done wrong. Nothing; it was just as we always did it. I draped again and he returned, tearing them off without saying a word. He entered the room for a third time and stated that I didn't want to help him.

"You don't even know how to drape the patient! Call Dr. Jimmy Howell, (a junior associate of Dr. DeBakey and a star yet to shine) and get him in here to help," he ordered. The next Monday when I scrubbed in the operating room, it got even worse.

"Dr. Diethrich, I've had enough of you. Go stand in the corner of the room and see if you can understand the sequences we are going through, and what we are trying to do with this patient." When I heard DeBakey say that to me, I knew it was over.

However, the harassment dragged on until I fell into a depression. I would return home late at night and tell Gloria, "This man is intentionally trying to break me. It's become a battle."

There were days when I would put on scrubs and fight down nausea at the very thought of going into surgery. I would go to Ed Garrett, Dr. DeBakey's senior surgeon, and ask for help. "Ed, I don't know how much more of this I can take. I'm losing my confidence; I dread walking into the operating room. And I've loved the operating room since I was fifteen."

I'd go to Jimmy Howell and beg him to scrub in and take my place. "I don't even want to be near it," Jimmy would say. It got so bad that in the lunchroom the anesthesiologists would comment, "Ted, don't come back in the operating room, you are not going to scrub again. You are on your way out of here." I was a person who had devoted so many years to becoming technically proficient, to achieving certain skills. To be ground down under DeBakey's heel was frightening.

Finally, I decided that I would not be beaten, even though when I looked in the mirror I wasn't sure which Ted I was seeing. In life, it's such moments as that, which offer a true perspective into one's inner character and strength. I began to understand that perseverance was my only option.

I was on the floor seeing patients when I received a page from Polly, saying Dr. DeBakey wanted me to go in Room #2 to expose the femoral artery for a femoral-popliteal bypass. He had three rooms: Room #2 was for peripheral and carotid, Room #3 was for heart, and Room #4 was for complex vascular procedures. He was in Room #3 with a heart case, so I went into Room #2 and exposed arteries at the groin and above the knee. At that time we were only using synthetic grafts for bypasses so I just waited, periodically inquiring how things in Room #3 were going. The nurse said it is getting worse by the moment. "The patient is on seventeen drips, and the doctor is throwing instruments around, cussing."

"Well, we will just stand by," I said. I looked up above to the dome where I had been during my interview. The fellows currently up there were motioning me to sew in the graft. These were my buddies, but I shook my head *no, no, no* that would surely be the end of me.

Every two minutes I asked the circulating nurse for a report from Room #3. After several of these brief conversations she ceased verbal communication, just shaking her head, indicating it was a disaster. Meanwhile, I would look up to the dome to see what the fellows were thinking. They had access to the dome in Room #3 and could get a quick picture of what was going on in there. I had no question about my ability to sew the graft in place; I had been sewing grafts for years.

After a repeat of this scenario several times, and another non-verbal report from the circulating nurse, I decided to put the graft in. My hands were as calm as always, and the nurse did not need to wipe any perspiration from my brow. There was none. I think the fellows upstairs had enough for all of us. My fear was the repercussions anticipated from Dr. DeBakey.

I sewed in the graft, and as always, after the graft was in place we put a needle distally and shot an on-the-table arteriogram. After the x-ray was developed I closed the incision and put the x-ray on the view box. Finally, he came in and looked at the incision.

"Dr. DeBakey, I put the bypass in and shot the angiogram. It's on the view box," I said. He walked over, looked at it, and then left the room without a word. I knew he was going to find Art Beall to have me discharged. Art was in charge of the fellows, and therefore the assassinator. I knew it.

At the close of the operating schedule I made rounds with DeBakey, but he didn't say anything. The next day we made rounds and things were seemingly okay, but I hadn't scrubbed back in again. I thought to myself, *I can't scrub or I'm surely out of here.* As we crossed the bridge with the usual legions of guys following, he abruptly stopped. Behind us came the domino effect, with all the fellows bumping into each other. He turned to me.

"Ted, starting tomorrow I want you to operate every day in Room #4."

I never knew what I had done to pass the test, because I never knew the rules of the test if indeed there were any. Sometime later Dr. DeBakey and I drove to Methodist Annex and were talking about a resident with whom the senior surgeon had been giving holy hell. Dr. DeBakey suddenly grew silent for a while, and his hands clutched the steering wheel tightly. He began to speak again in a flat, cold voice.

"Ted, you know, I test people. I see what people can do under fire and under pressure. I must know what these people are made of."

Apparently my endurance under the fire and pressure satisfied him because after assigning me to Room #4 my life changed from night to day. My relationship with Dr. DeBakey was entirely different; he began gradually treating me more like an associate. Oh, it was not always calm and peaceful, but the stress now was related to our work. He literally gave me anything I requested. The new research laboratory was completely open to any work my colleagues and I wanted to do, and most important- ly, it was funded. I cannot recall one request I made that did not receive a positive response. It

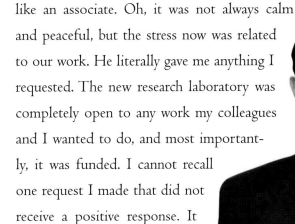

Survival test passed.

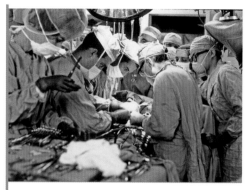

The high pressure zone.

became a fertile environment in which a young cardiovascular surgeon could learn and mature.

Dr. DeBakey was very busy with his practice and the duties at the school. Due to his international reputation, he was constantly being asked to speak or meet representatives from companies, and more often than not he would tell Polly to have me see what they wanted. Who knew that one of those meetings would be a little bit life changing?

The gentleman was tall, casually dressed, and carrying a notebook. He introduced himself as Thomas Thompson, otherwise known as Tommy Thompson, a writer for *LIFE* magazine. He wanted to talk to Dr. DeBakey about heart surgery and was particularly interested in heart transplantation.

We immediately struck up a conversation because this was one of my particular areas of research. I told Dr. DeBakey about our visit, and he said he would meet Tommy when it was convenient. I am not sure if his interview ever occurred, but Tommy and I became very close friends. He learned to play frontenis (more on that later), came to my house on the weekends when many of the young staff and fellows were relaxing, went skiing in Aspen with me and my Michigan friends; in short, he actually became a member of our family during his frequent visits to Houston.

His book *Hearts* was literally written at our dining room table where we spent many evenings discussing what he was observing and learning from his interviews at the medical center. Published in 1971 as a nonfiction account of the rivalry between DeBakey and Cooley, *Hearts* was part of a string of successful books by Tommy. Some of the material in *SLED* references his book *Hearts*.

Unfortunately, Tommy faced an early death but not before he wrote a second book *Blood and Money*. I had not read it in years until Tommy's son Kirk called and relayed that he and his brother Scott, were working on the filming of this book.

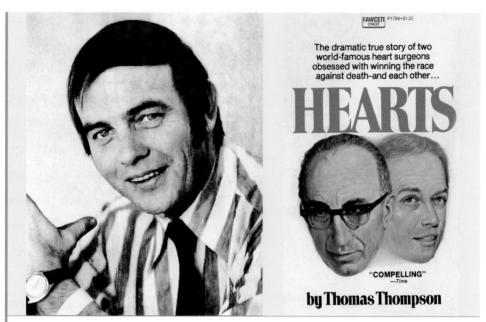

Thomas Thompson and his book *Hearts*.

The story is about Dr. John Hill, the baritone player in the "Heartbeats" Band (an all physician band directed by Dr. Cooley's associate, Dr. Grady Hallman). In 1969 an assassin, presumably contracted by John Hill himself, murdered his wife in their Houston home. The assumption was that the father-in-law then put a contract out on John Hill. It will be a fascinating movie, but it is unlikely that any of the "Heartbeat" rhythms will be incorporated into the sound track.

Of the many visitors that Dr. DeBakey asked me to greet and tour, Tommy Thompson was from several aspects the most important. We developed a family friendship which lasts today with his two sons. However, from a professional aspect, the meeting with Dr. Hans Moore, an executive of Philips & Co. in Europe, turned out to be a real game changer for not only me but the entire development of the endovascular specialty. Hans greeted me with the question, "Dr. Diethrich, what is the greatest need you see in the future for radiographic equipment?" He hit the center of the bullseye. This was my all-consuming issue. If we were to develop the potential for endovascular therapy, it could not be done with fixed equipment and a snap shot photo like the one I did for Dr.

*To Ted & Gloria —
Without whom this
would never have
happened —
Thanks & love —*

Thomas Thompson

DeBakey to show the functioning femoral popliteal bypass.

I was already working with Drs. Marty Kaplitt and Phil Sawyer from Long Island, NY on a procedure called CO_2 gas endarterectomy. The technique was simple but effective. CO_2 gas was passed through a fine needle and introduced into the obstructed artery. The gas expanded the outer arterial lining and the arthroscopic core could be extracted. What was needed was an angiogram to confirm the flow beyond the obstruction after the artery was cleared. It required the same technique as the cardiologists were using in coronary arteriography and angioplasty. I explained this to Hans in detail. His response was as simple as my question. "Dr. Diethrich, we do not have that type of equipment for the operating room at the present time." "Can we get it?" I replied. Sorry, very doubtful, it is not in the pipeline of our new product development. I dropped the subject, deeply discouraged. I knew that precise angiography equipment would be essential in our future work.

A week before I was to move on to the next residency training rotation, a big surprise occurred. Ed Garrett came to me and said that Dr. DeBakey didn't want me to rotate. He wanted me to stay on his service there at Methodist Hospital.

Stop the presses!

From washing instruments as a sixteen-year-old high school student to an invitation to join the team of the world's leading vascular surgeon—that was quite a headline story for a fellow who, only months earlier, was having trouble looking in the mirror, expecting his career to end at any moment.

9

Science Fiction
Meets Special Ops

All over the world, interest in cardiac transplantation was increasing. It occurred to me that one of the roadblocks in our progress might be finding a proper transport to support the donor to the recipient's site and prolong the viability of the heart until transplantation.

My resident, John Liddicoat, and I worked in the school research laboratory alongside Dr. DeBakey's artificial heart program team directed by Bill Hall and Domingo Liotta. I had developed a relationship with Grumman Aerospace Corporation, which allowed engineers to work and investigate the potential to preserve the heart while awaiting transplantation. The idea was to remove both heart and lungs from a donor, put them into a chamber (about the size of a dishwasher), bathe them with a cooling mist, and keep them under constant monitoring. This would preserve them alive and healthy until they could be transplanted into a recipient. The chamber also had to be small and portable, so it could be flown anywhere in the world.

Several dog hearts had been kept alive for more than thirty hours, and on one occasion, in late 1969, a human heart had lived within the chamber for almost two days. As a test, we even chartered a Lear jet and flew the chamber to retrieve organs from a San Antonio hospital. It was a success. To see the suspended organs pulsating within the chamber—the heart beating from its natural pacemaker, seemingly floating in the mist—was reminiscent of a horror film.

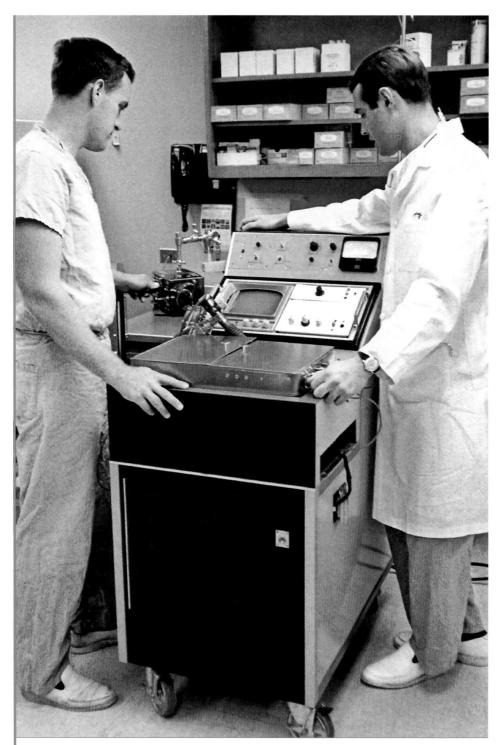

John Liddicoat and me working with the preservation chamber constructed by Grumman Aerospace Corporation.

I took a lot of kidding as Dr. Frankenstein, but I saw the project in a different light: it was outer-space medicine.

The annual American Medical Association's scientific exhibit session seemed like the ideal place to demonstrate our work. The meeting was held at the McCormick Center near Lake Michigan in Chicago. The committee invited members to submit abstracts that described the nature of their scientific work for the competition. We were already very active in competitions involving surgical motion pictures, winning almost every challenge available.

This Chicago opportunity seemed perfect to demonstrate our Preservation Chamber. The real excitement for the exhibit was the fact that we would have the chamber *operational*, meaning the heart and lungs would be visible with a heart beating and lungs expanding. In short: "It's alive!"

Can you imagine the logistical nightmare of this endeavor? We were in Houston at Baylor with the Preservation Chamber and its ancillary equipment, and the exhibit place was a three-hour flight north to Chicago.

I contacted my friend, Dr. Constantine (Dino) Tatooles, to help make the arrangements. (I had met Dino when he visited Houston as a Coller scholar, and we became immediate buddies. Dino became an outstanding surgeon, the youngest to ever have the chairmanship of the heart surgery department at Cook County Hospital in Chicago.) We would need a canine patient and an operating room to remove the heart and lungs before placing them in the Preservation Chamber. A respirator was required to support the pulmonary function, and glucose and calcium would be required for the heart function. Then, once in the chamber, we would need a support vehicle to transport the chamber to the exhibit hall.

Dino and I spent considerable time planning the exercise. Well, it wasn't nearly what it took for the human multiple organ transplantation venture, but more on that later in Chapter 14. We arrived a day early and set up everything in the laboratory at the University of Illinois where Dino had an appointment as Chief of Cardiac Surgery.

On the day of the procedure, we all arrived early in the experimental operating room. We had performed the procedure at least 50 times and were sure it would go well. Timing, however, was a major factor. We had to arrive at McCormick Center just prior to when the judging panel would be approaching our exhibit. That would assure our ability to explain the chamber to them personally. We used an ambulance as our transportation, just in case we were running late and needed a siren to get through traffic.

So far everything was progressing smoothly, except for a line checking the blood pressure that had come loose. For a few seconds, blood was spurting out all over the place, but we rapidly reconnected the line. As we pulled up to the exhibit entrance of the Center, we opened the rear doors and began to remove the chamber.

Two very large men approached me, one of them shouting, "What do you think you're doing?" I explained that I was Dr. Diethrich from Houston, and we were moving the chamber into the exhibit hall. It seemed like a very logical explanation to me until he screamed abruptly, "Where are your union papers?"

Obviously I had no union credentials. Doctors had no unions, and certainly no cards to permit equipment transfer. It was obvious to me that the fellows were not about to be receptive to discussion or negotiation. But I was on a time clock, and it was not the union one. If we did not get the chamber into the exhibit space soon, there would be no chance in the competition. I would have failed.

But suddenly I thought of Dino and had a glimmer of hope in my mind. I went to the pay phone and dialed my friend. It was the briefest phone communication I have ever had with him. "Ted, hang up," he instructed. Had I failed again with this idea?

I looked at my watch. Time was ticking away. I was explaining the situation to my crew, especially my resident, John Liddicoat, when suddenly out of nowhere appeared three of the biggest, blackest limousines I had ever seen. They came to a screeching halt next to the ambulance, and every limo deployed troops. The obvious leader shouted, "Who is Dr. Detwhich?" I stepped forward, but before I could identify myself or perhaps even shake hands he asked, "What is the problem here?"

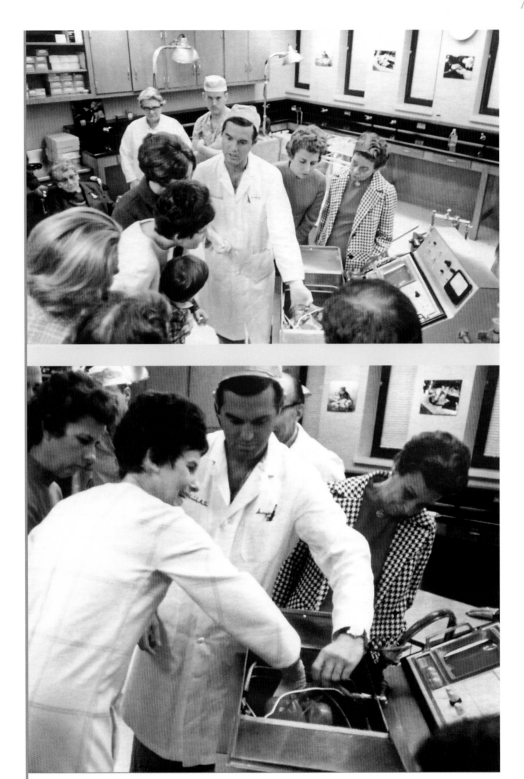

First models of the preservation chamber.

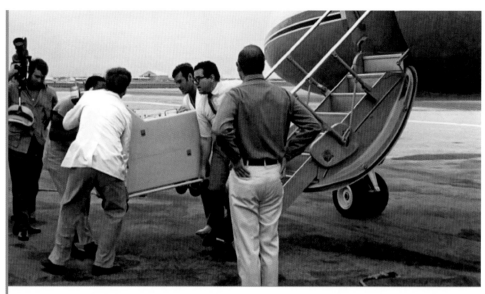

The portable chamber created maximum flexibility for transporting donor organs.

"These folks won't let us take the equipment into the exhibit hall." I replied as quickly as possible.

"Stand aside," he ordered. His gang immediately moved the chamber to our space in the hall. There was no conversation. It was like we didn't speak the same language. I had never been introduced to the Mafia, but it didn't matter; he already knew his assignment.

Incredibly, we were able to get all the lines and chamber connections completed just as the judges were leaving the adjacent exhibit. As they entered our space, I stood there as a proud scientific exhibitor at the AMA Annual Convention. The judges would never know what it took to pull this whole thing off, but they were really impressed. Perhaps they thought they were seeing a scene from science fiction.

Yes, we won first place and the highest honor, the Hektoen Gold Medal Award. I was very proud when Dr. DeBakey congratulated me upon my return to Houston.

Much more important, however, were the words I recalled when I told Dr. Coller years before that I had received the DeBakey appointment: "Young boy, today you learned a great lesson. It's not what you know, but who." A lesson repeated. Thanks again, Dino.

10

Black Mike and the Bubble Oxygenator

In the Cooley camp there were continuous disparaging remarks regarding Dr. DeBakey at Methodist. Frequently, he was referred to as "Black Mike." I never understood why or the origin of the name, but it did trouble me.

My transition from the research laboratories at Baylor College of Medicine to the operating rooms of Methodist and St. Luke's Hospitals across the street was an easy exercise…One day it was with a dog, then a pig, then a sheep, and then on to the *Homo sapiens*. That, of course, is an exaggeration, but many times what I observed in the lab was soon to be tested in the clinical setting.

An example of this was the total artificial heart. I frequently went to St. Luke's to observe Dr. Cooley and his team at work. Dr. Art Beall, the man referred to earlier as the executioner when a resident had to be fired, was very active in developing the disposable bubble oxygenator. A product of the Travenol Laboratories in Morton Grove, Illinois, this development changed open-heart surgery overnight.

With the conventional oxygenator, a large volume of blood was required, as well as excessive time in cleaning and sterilization. This limited the number of cases that could be performed.

However, with the disposable bubble oxygenator, thirty or more patients could have heart surgery per day. I was anxious to see this new equipment used on humans after having observed the animal studies next door. It was really quite phenomenal.

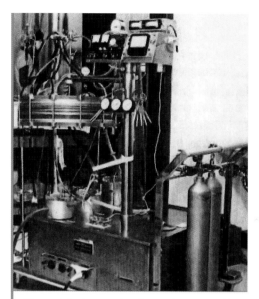

The original complex heart lung machine, requiring large amounts of blood for priming.

As one famous British surgeon, Mr. Donald Ross (in the UK, surgeons are addressed as Mr.), commented after visiting an operation using the bubble oxygenator: "I was devastated. The by-pass was switched on, and I swear the atrial septal defect was closed before the oxygenated blood ever reached the femoral artery. A mass of foam emerged like a chimney stack from the top of the oxygenator, but by then Denton Cooley was in his cab on the way to the airport to report his 1000 cases."

One day, after watching Dr. Cooley replace a valve using the disposable bubble oxygenator, I left St. Luke's and headed back to Methodist to make rounds with Dr. DeBakey. I explained my excitement for this new technology, and he acknowledged that it had great potential.

As we moved from room to room, I told Dr. DeBakey I was troubled by something. The reference to Black Mike I had heard at St. Luke's seemed extraordinarily disrespectful to me. Dr. DeBakey stopped and turned to me.

"Ted, whenever you are climbing the ladder toward success there will always be people nipping at your feet. As long as your mission is laudable, just keep on climbing. They will eventually fall far behind."

That lesson stayed with me the rest of my career.

11

A Matter of the Heart–
Stolen or Just Substituted?

Thousands of words have been written on this subject by hundreds of authors, some with prejudice, some with first-hand information, but most with speculations. The subject I am referring to is the artificial heart that was transplanted into the chest of Haskell Karp at St. Luke's Hospital in Houston, Texas, on April 4, 1969, by Dr. Denton A. Cooley and Dr. Domingo S. Liotta, a cardiac surgeon from Argentina. What gives me the credentials to opine on this event?

I believe I might be one of only a few who know the true story of the "stolen" heart, which is how it was often referred to in later publications.

Earlier in this book, I referenced my work with the preservation chamber and canine heart transplantation experiments with Dr. John Liddicoat. This work was done in the laboratories at Baylor College of Medicine, right across the street from the Methodist and St. Luke's Hospitals.

Directly next to the lab where we worked was a second lab, where Dr. DeBakey's artificial heart team was busy

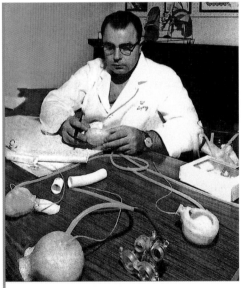

Domingo Liotta, MD, shown with his artificial heart creation.

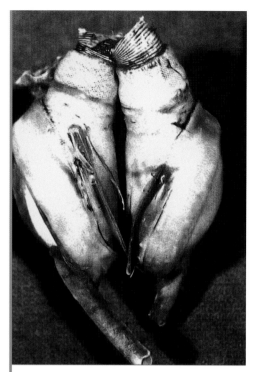

There were two separate pumps representing the right and left side of the heart.

implanting the mechanical device into calves. Dr. Domingo Liotta was the leader of that team, assisted by William Hall, and the clinical cardiopulmonary pump team for both St. Luke's and Methodist Hospitals. Within the clinical pump technician team, Mary Martin and "Euford" were the mainstays.

John was in the lab much more frequently than I, but at the very least I dropped in every few days or so, poked my head into the calf laboratory, and inquired about how their artificial heart project was progressing. I never encountered Dr. Cooley or his associates on any of my visits.

Over all, I had a feeling that the "team" was looking forward to a clinical application. It wasn't uncommon to hear comments like, "We don't know what it is going to take to convince the old man (again referring to Dr. DeBakey) to try it out." These were the usual positives and negatives associated with every research activity.

On the morning of April 4, 1969, Dr. DeBakey flew to Washington, DC, where he had to testify to the National Institutes of Health (NIH) regarding the artificial heart transplantation program at Baylor College of Medicine. With Dr. DeBakey out of town, our service at Methodist was slow that day. I had gone to my son Tad's football practice, and upon arriving home I turned on the TV to get the news. I did not expect the report I saw.

It was a view of the operating room at St. Luke's Hospital, alongside an announcement that Dr. Denton Cooley had just implanted an artificial heart. I could not believe my eyes or ears—that just could not have happened. I quickly called John and told him to meet me at Methodist Hospital. We changed into scrubs and walked through the tunnel to the St. Luke's operating room.

There, in the middle of the operating theatre, was a patient on a respirator connected to the artificial heart pumps I had seen across the street. Several monitors were analyzing pressure, flow, blood gases, and the patients' electrocardiogram (ECG). Domingo greeted us with a friendly smile.

"What do you think, Ted?"

It was a good thing I had a surgical mask on, because my disbelief at this initial comment would have been patently obvious. I asked a few questions about the pumps, noting that the patient seemed to be very stable. Suddenly, Dr. Cooley came into the room; he had probably just completed another operation.

"How's it look, Ted?"

"Seems pretty successful to me, Denton. What is the plan?" was my reply.

"We'll support him with this until a donor heart becomes available, hopefully soon."

"Congratulations and good luck. I'll see you later," I commented, still feeling amazed at what I was witnessing. John and I walked back through the tunnel to Methodist Hospital. We were in a state of shock. In fact, we could have used a little of that cardiac support ourselves.

Beyond acknowledging the magnitude of what we had just observed, my mind was fixed on the next step. Dr. Cooley was my mentor and friend, but I was Dr. DeBakey's associate. He was most likely sound asleep at the Hayes Hotel in DC, awaiting the next morning's encounter with the congressmen on the artificial heart program.

Of course, at that point in time I had no idea what Dr. Liotta would reveal about the transplant several years later in his dissertation below:

In the afternoon of April 4, Denton—still working in the OR1—asked Dr. Bob Leachman to call Dr. DeBakey to inform him of what was going on at the Texas Heart Institute. Unfortunately, Mike was already flying to Washington; and the worst thing was the fact that the following morning Dr. DeBakey entered the room at the NIH meeting in Washington and received the warm congratulations on the artificial heart implantation by the NIH members.

Even though Dr. Liotta published that in 2012, it was exactly what was pressing on my mind in 1969. In good conscious, I could not allow Dr. DeBakey to go to the committee without this knowledge.

I drove home fast. (As I write this now, I think, *how did we live without cell phones?*) I knew it was the middle of the night in Washington, but I dialed the hotel and asked for his room. Several rings, then a tired-sounding "hello?"

"Dr. DeBakey, this is Ted. I have something very important to tell you before your meeting in the morning. Are you awake?"

"Yes, go ahead." I told the tale of what I had encountered in as much detail as possible. I made it clear that it was the Baylor Research Team led by Dr. Cooley who performed the artificial heart implantation. "Do you understand?"

"Yes, thank you," he replied. The line went dead.

I am quite certain that if I had not made that phone call, Dr. DeBakey could have been completely broadsided and embarrassed the next morning. Possibly someone else might have called, but it was very unlikely. Dr. Liotta's later account regarding Dr. Leachman does not seem entirely realistic to me.

As friendly as I was with Denton Cooley, I never discussed the total artificial heart episode with him. I just assumed the total artificial heart I had observed that day in St Luke's operating room was the same I had seen in the laboratory at Baylor College of Medicine. The same one referred to as "Dr. DeBakey's artificial heart," for which he had received a grant from the NIH in 1964. The grant was for the collaborative Baylor/Rice artificial heart program; Rice was selected because of its outstanding capabilities in engineering.

Prior to writing this particular chapter, I read the published accounts of the investigative studies by Domingo Liotta and more recently the book *100,000 Hearts* by Dr. Denton A. Cooley. The account he published in 2012 presents

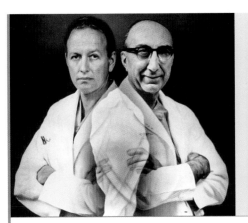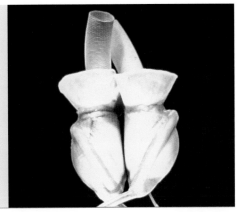

Dr. Denton Cooley, left, and Dr. Michael DeBakey, right, when the controversy was ignited due to the confusion of whose artificial heart was actually implanted.

an entirely different perspective on this drama, in which Dr. Domingo Liotta was a key actor.

In Cooley's book, Domingo was offered a surgical fellowship by Dr. DeBakey to work on what he thought would be his (Domingo's) total artificial heart. However, Dr. DeBakey's interests shifted toward left ventricular assist devices, which could help support a failing heart. According to Dr. Liotta, his artificial heart (the one reported in the 1961 literature) was not receiving Dr. DeBakey's enthusiasm.

Domingo felt that Dr. DeBakey would never try it, and out of frustration, he met with Dr. Cooley at St. Luke's Hospital in December 1968. Dr. Cooley agreed to work with Domingo on the Liotta total artificial heart. Financial assistance was included. This was all conducted in conjunction with Rice and Dr. J. David Holland, who was also a collaborator of Dr. DeBakey's Baylor/Rice total artificial heart program.

The only thing required by Dr. Cooley was that Bill O'Bannon, the engineer who was to build the control console, would not allow this project to interfere with his normal work. Therefore, Bill did the construction in his home workshop. After extensive bench tests and seven implants in the calves, it was decided the device was ready, but only to be used in a desperate situation, the condition they had agreed upon at the onset of their combined work.

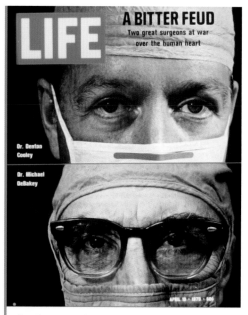

"Stolen Heart" *LIFE* magazine cover.

The initial operation was done on April 4, 1969, and the recipient was Haskell Karp. After the total artificial heart implantation, he went on to have a cardiac transplantation by Dr. Cooley, but did not survive due to infection and weakness of the immune system. He died on April 8, just thirty-two hours after the heart transplant.

Dr. Cooley described the turmoil this operation created for him. It led to censorship by the American College of Surgeons, dismissal from the University professorship, extensive negative press and more. However, he survived it all and went on to create the world-renowned Texas Heart Institute. The major controversy was centered around which heart was actually inserted.

It is important to appreciate that the actual artificial heart, which has two parts, a left and a right, is within the chest cavity. Not visible! The two pumps outside the chest are connected to the heart by tubes, again one for the right and the other for the left. So it is not possible to know what the artificial heart inside the chest looks like just by observing the pumps.

My thinking initially was that it was the DeBakey total artificial heart, but you see, in all actuality there were two separate artificial hearts. Since it was not my experiment, it would not be apparent to me with simple, quick periodic observations in the calf laboratory. Plus, the personnel were all the same in the laboratory—Liotta, Hall, and the pump team from Methodist and St. Luke's Hospitals. Of course, then there is the key question: What authority and administrative body granted permission to the surgeon to perform this experimental operation? That was a huge complex question, all a part of the overall investigation.

Dr. DeBakey's artificial heart program was supported by the NIH grant, while Dr. Liotta's was funded primarily by Dr. Cooley. In the first scenario, Dr. Cooley would have been obligated to obtain permission for the procedure; under the second scenario, perhaps not.

On the other hand, Rice University personnel constructed the Liotta artificial heart, the same people who were supported by an NIH grant for their work on Dr. DeBakey's artificial heart and the partial heart bypass products. Furthermore, the animal experimentation occurred in the Baylor laboratories.

With these facts known, it's clear that I am perhaps the one to opine on this story after all. From what I am able to gather, the heart placed in Mr. Karp was not the Dr. DeBakey heart defined as a Baylor product. It was the total artificial heart that Dr. Domingo Liotta reported in the *Transactions of the American Society for Artificial Organs* in 1961 (Volume 7, pages 318–322).

Dr. DeBakey and Dr. Cooley did not speak to each other for more than forty years because of this situation. Finally, on May 2, 2008, they shook hands when Dr. Cooley was given honorary membership into the Michael E. DeBakey International Society and a lifetime achievement award.

An excerpt from the 2010 book *Open Heart* also reveals some different accounts of the stolen heart story, since author David K.C. Cooper, MD, interviewed Dr. DeBakey while writing it. In the book, according to Dr. DeBakey:

> "The man who was partly responsible for this was working in my laboratory as an assistant technician (referring to Domingo Liotta, later to become a well-known surgeon in South America). He was Argentinean. To the committee that had to investigate this matter, he said that he felt I would refuse to use our device on human beings, and he was quite correct. I was opposed to using it on humans because we couldn't get survival in our animals for more than a few months. They all died. We couldn't figure out why, or how to prevent that. I didn't feel that ethically we could go to an institutional review board and get

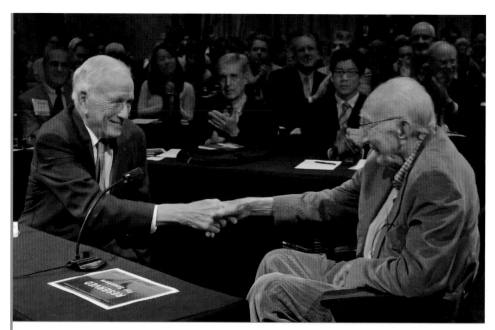

Forty years later, the great mentors reunite. Photograph courtesy of Baylor College of Medicine Archives.

approval for the device to be used as an experimental procedure on humans. So, secretly, he went to Dr. Cooley and discussed this with him. I'm not sure yet whether he or Dr. Cooley initiated it, but the fact remains that they got together secretly and agreed they would do it.

So, one night, he removed the artificial heart from our laboratory and brought it over to Dr. Cooley. They had it all organized. This happened when I was out of town. They had this patient with an aneurysm of the left ventricle (a weakening and dilation of the ventricle resulting from the presence of dead muscle following a heart attack). They scheduled it as a resection of ventricular aneurysm, but they knew they were going to use the artificial heart; they had the device there (in the operating room). They had hardly gotten started with the operation when he (Dr. Cooley) said to remove the patient's heart. So they did. The device was implanted. It was publicized tremendously," continued DeBakey.

"You can't help but wonder how it got so publicized. They had obviously called the press to tell them they were going to do it. I was in Washington, and as I went to bed that night and happened to turn on the television in the hotel, there it was on the news. It was a shock. I was at a meeting at the NIH and so, when I got to the NIH the next morning, they asked me about it. I said, "I didn't know anything about it." It created a serious problem, because all of our work was supported by the NIH. We had to explain to them how this had been done when it hadn't been approved by them or by the hospital review board."

Maybe Dr. DeBakey forgot my late night call? He did sound sleepy, but I was sure my message to him created a sleeper's nightmare.

Regardless of the various scenarios and who said what to whom, the consequences were enormous. I believe Dr. DeBakey immediately called his sisters, Lois and Selma. They were medical writers, and I worked frequently on scientific papers with them. The reason I believe he contacted them is clear, because over a very short period of time, the world was notified of what became known as the "stolen heart story."

It was a key topic of discussion in every place I traveled in the U.S. and abroad. Dr. Cooley was discharged from Baylor and disciplined as could have been anticipated. He never missed a beat and continued to be one of the finest cardiac surgeons in the world. Other members of the team went about their way as the flames of the fire died.

However, it was apparent that the Department of Surgery at Baylor College of Medicine had changed forever.

12

Introduction to Europe— The Beginning of Opportunities

A lot of whispered talk was going on in the operating rooms. Apparently, Dr. DeBakey was planning a large trip to Europe. It was not uncommon for him to go overseas for short periods of time to lecture, but this seemed different. The plan was to take a full operating team, heart-lung equipment, and all supporting materials for multiple operations in several countries.

He had not discussed the plan with me personally, but the OR supervisor Dana Estes, RN, was fully aware of it, and August dates were proposed. In late June, Ed Garrett came into my office and closed the door. Ed never closed the door. That was a bad sign.

"Ted, the old man is planning a big operating trip to Europe. I have not told him yet, but I am not going." I was shocked. Ed was Dr. DeBakey's senior associate, whom he always called when there was a problem. He was a solid fixture of the operating team.

Ed said his decision was related to a new valve Dr. DeBakey was developing with a US company. We had put several of the valves in over the past months, and Ed was almost always part of the procedure. He had reviewed the data, followed up on the patients, and found there was an excessive incidence of hemolysis, which is a breakdown of red blood cells. The cause was not certain, but there was suspicion that the cobalt ball of the caged-ball prosthesis was the culprit since it had not been used in other valves.

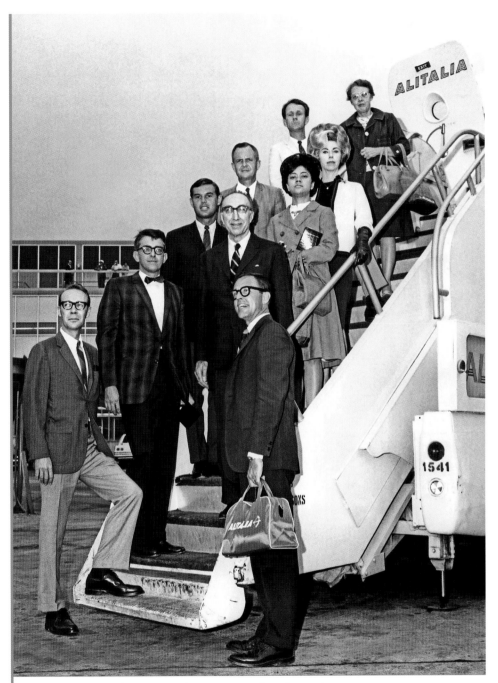

Houston team deplaning at Malpensa Airport in Milan, Italy.

Top to bottom: Mary Martin, head of the pump team; Ellen Morris, scrub RN; Euford Martin; Gracie Soto, scrub RN; Ed Dennis, MD; Michael DeBakey, MD; Edward Diethrich, MD; James Fenstermacher, MD; Lyal Williams, MD anesthesiologist; and Wayne Ulrich, Administrative Assistant.

Ed was very disturbed by the results and felt the use of the valve should be suspended pending further engineering assessment. Dr. DeBakey was not of the mood to accept that decision and planned on using the valve during the upcoming European operating trip. Ed felt he could not in good conscience go with the team, perhaps contributing to a problem of hemolysis in foreign countries. There was no changing his mind. He was going to tell Dr. DeBakey later in the day, and he suggested that I take his place.

On one hand, I would be a poorly qualified substitute for Ed Garrett on such an important trip; on the other, what an opportunity! I thought briefly about the ethical issue of a poorly functioning valve, but clearly that was out of my pay grade level of decision-making. Dr. DeBakey would make those decisions independently.

By the end of the discussion, I had a feeling there was more to the issue than just a valve. Maybe Ed was thinking of moving on. It was just a few hours later when Dr. DeBakey came to see me, explaining that Ed was not going to Europe and I would be part of the team.

After I thanked him, he immediately gave me a list of lectures and movies he wanted for the trip. Almost all of them were new, which meant I would have to work around the clock with the audiovisual (AV) department if we were to meet the schedule. Right away I called Herb Smith, head of the AV department, and we started preparations that evening.

The plane from Houston landed in Milan, Italy, at the new Malpensa Airport. I am not sure how many flights had landed at this new airport; we might have been the first. Either way, everything seemed well organized.

It was about ten o'clock in the morning when officials boarded the plane and greeted Dr. DeBakey. The plan was for Dr. DeBakey, the cardiologist Ed Dennis, the anesthesiologists and me to go directly to the University of Milan. The rest of the team would be transported to the hotel for some rest.

At the University we were seated in a classical European-style amphitheatre, where the residents gave the potential patient presentations to Dr. DeBakey. Ed Dennis and I were seated behind Dr. DeBakey and Professor Milan, who was our host. We

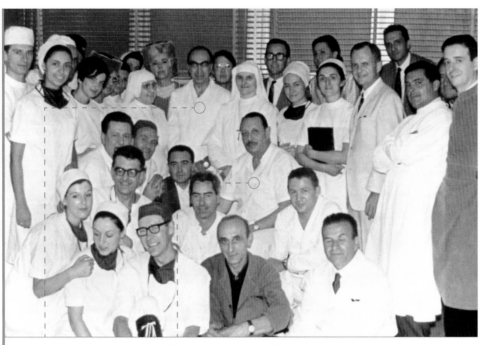

Dr. DeBakey with Professor Milan at the center of the operating team.

paid special attention to each case, as Dr. DeBakey would nod his head, indicating whether he would accept the patient for operation or not. Ed and I, along with the anesthesiologists, compiled our list and ultimately put the operating schedule together.

Without that careful selection it would have been a disaster. They had several very ill patients who were categorized as high risk for surgery—even for our OR team in Houston. There were press everywhere, daily headlines in the paper, and Dr. DeBakey proudly speaking of modern cardiovascular surgery achievements. Only one cobalt valve was used in Milan without an acute incident, but of course that was not the real test; only time would tell, and Ed Garrett knew that.

Even with the best plans and details worked out in advance, an endeavor of this magnitude was subject to unexpected events. Such was the case of a patient who required a mitral valve replacement. The operation went well; however, in the ICU we noted more than usual drainage from the chest tubes. I was keeping a very close eye on the situation and updating Dr. DeBakey every hour or so even though the patient was very stable.

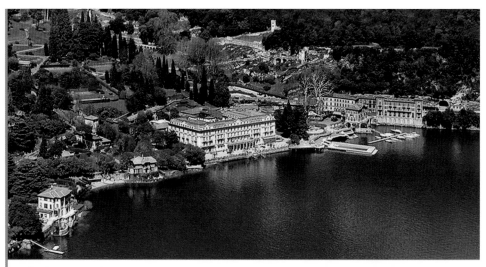

Villa d'Este Hotel

When he came to the bedside late in the afternoon he said that Prof. Milan and his staff had planned a dinner event in our honor at the Villa d'Este Hotel on Lake Como that evening. He said that he felt compelled to stay with the patient and that I should go in his place and represent the Houston team. In turn, I suggested that I stay with the patient and he attend the dinner, but he was not receptive to that suggestion. I went to Lake Como with no idea of what to expect. Of course, this was the very first of what would later be numerous trips to Italy, and the initiation of my European operating experience. In the future I would operate throughout Europe several times a year.

The Villa d'Este Hotel was spectacular on the shore of the lake. George Clooney today has a beautiful home not far from the hotel. In fact, years later I revisited the region with Gloria and Thelma Kieckhefer from the Arizona Heart Foundation Board.

In Dr. DeBakey's absence I was obligated to give a thank you speech on behalf of our team. However, under my breath I was saying a private thank you to DeBakey for this wonderful experience.

It would have been wonderful if I could have ended my visit to Milan that evening, but the next day Dr. DeBakey was to perform a renal artery bypass. That's when a graft is sutured to the aorta, and then to the artery feeding the kidney to bypass an obstruction. I dreaded helping Dr. DeBakey on the procedure. It seemed he was not so comfortable with the operation, and in fact back in Houston it was Dr. George Morris who was the expert on renal bypass operations. Dr. DeBakey sutured the bypass and I assisted. He always packed 4x4 gauze around the suture sites to promote clotting of the needle holes.

After about five minutes when the bypass was functioning, Dr. DeBakey told me to clear the anastomosis (the area of the suturing). I removed the gauze and placed my index finger on the renal artery to check the pulse. There was a brisk bleed coming from the distal end of the graft. Really, it was more than brisk; the blood was welling up.

Dr. DeBakey had turned to answer some questions from a visiting surgeon, and then he turned and saw the bleeding. He accused me of creating a problem by examining the artery with my finger. It was nonsense, but as always I never said a word. After all, there were visitors and press everywhere.

I kept my finger on the bleeding site like the Dutch boy plugging the hole in the dike to prevent a flood. We fixed the problem, but I was really angry about the episode. He was blaming me for something that was not my fault.

From Milan our team moved to Yugoslavia, where our first stop was Lubiana, otherwise known as Ljubljana. After a busy work week, everyone went to the mountains on Saturday for a festive picnic. Their team was extremely friendly, and I kept in touch for many years. It was here I had my first introduction to Slivovitz, a brandy made from local plums. From there we went to Zagreb (the capital of Croatia), and finally Belgrade (the capital of Serbia).

As we moved from west to east, the varying levels of sophistication became more obvious. I'm not referring to the physicians on staff, but rather the vintage of equipment and certain protocols such as sterility.

For example, on that first day in Zagreb the operating room was all set. I was about to make the sternal incision, when suddenly the circulating nun appeared next to the instrument table, abruptly lifted a fly swatter, and whacked a fly that had landed on the instrument stand. She was a good shot. The fly lay dead with outstretched wings, right next to the scalpel I was about to use.

The most troubling example was in the Belgrade military hospital. We were finishing an aortic valve replacement with the cobalt valve. After re-warming the patient, the heart came back to the usual ventricular fibrillation pattern (meaning an irregular, ineffective rhythm), which required a defibrillator machine in order to convert to a normal action. It is not unlike what we see in our airports every day now. I called for the defibrillator. The circulating nurse informed me there was none in the hospital, and they would have to go across town to obtain one. It might take an hour or so, which meant an extra hour on the heart lung machine.

In my lab at St. Joseph's we often encountered ventricular fibrillation in our operations. Before I convinced the Head Sister to provide us with a used defibrillator machine, I had a makeshift method that worked. I would take an extension cord, strip the outer cover away for a short distance, and tape the bare wires to two large spoons that were attached to tongue blades with adhesive tape. This was the defibrillator paddle assembly. The extension cord was pushed into the wall socket when the electrical shock was to be delivered and then quickly withdrawn. Crude as it seemed, it worked, and no one was ever electrocuted.

I had dropped out of scrub at the operating table and was desperately preparing my homemade defibrillator paddles. The nun and the hospital engineer were running around feverishly to assist me. As luck would have it, the defibrillator from across town arrived at about the same time my substitute device was ready. The patient made an uneventful recovery, and we were all looking forward to returning to Methodist Hospital in Houston.

13

From Acapulco to Arizona—
A Frontenis Affair

In the mid 1960s, there seemed to be a very high volume of carotid endarterectomy cases at the Methodist Hospital. The purpose of this particular operation was to remove plaque in the carotid artery, purportedly to reduce the risk of stroke.

Dr. John McCutchen was a young neurologist on staff at the hospital. He spent most of his time seeing Dr. DeBakey's patients due to the high prevalence of these cases. To this day, there continues a debate about the value of the operation and who should and should not have it.

There were also early debates about who did the first carotid endarterectomy procedure. In the U.S., Dr. DeBakey received the credit. In Europe, it was Mr. Ian Eastcott at St. Mary's Hospital in London. Regardless, I am sure Dr. DeBakey did many more procedures than his European colleague.

John McCutchen and I became close friends while working on Dr. DeBakey's service. One day he introduced me to Mr. Gutierrez, a patient from Mexico who wanted to invite us to Acapulco for a long weekend. I later learned he had been Mexico's Secretary of the Treasury.

We arrived in Acapulco late in the evening and were picked up by a driver sent by Mr. Gutierrez. His home was on the far west side, high on a hill overlooking the Pacific Ocean. By the time we settled in, it was too late and dark to really appreciate the magnitude and beauty of the villa.

The next morning I was up early for my usual run, and as I surveyed the grounds over a porch rail, I saw some kind of sport court. It had three walls; a front, left side and back, with no wall on the right. Mr. Gutierrez' son saw me craning my neck for a better view and came up to explain the structure to me.

"It is a fronton court. We play using specially strung tennis rackets and rubber balls made in Mexico City. We call the sport frontenis. There are over 2000 courts in Mexico City alone."

Within ten minutes I was in my game shorts and on the court for my first frontenis lesson, which I called "fronton" for short from then on. I had played tennis, handball, racquetball, and squash, but they were no match for the three-walled sport on the fronton court.

We played singles and doubles to exhaustion. I did not want to leave Acapulco, and on the plane home I discussed with Gloria the idea of buying a house in Houston and constructing a fronton. She was less than lukewarm about the idea. It did not matter. I was hooked! So, we bought an old house on the west side of Houston with enough surrounding property to accommodate the new fronton court.

An official court is 100 feet long, but due to available land, mine was to be 60 feet long, thirty feet high and thirty feet wide. Construction began and the walls were taking shape. Gloria was focused on designing the inside of the old house, barely paying any attention to my project.

We were three-quarters of the way finished with the court when I left town on a Wednesday to speak in Chicago. Right after landing, I received an urgent message from my secretary. The neighbor across the street was threatening a lawsuit with an injunction to stop construction of the court immediately. According to the legal papers, "It was too high, too ugly, and it was disruptive to the natural surroundings of the neighborhood." He was demanding that we tear it down.

I gave my presentation the following day and caught the next flight back to Houston. I instructed my secretary to get the contractor at the house for an urgent meeting upon my arrival. We met late Thursday evening, and I was prepared with a plan. If he could put a full court press into completing all the walls over the weekend, I might be able to divert the angry neighbor across the driveway. The contractor agreed, and a frantic construction of concrete blocks ensued. Unbeknownst to me, the neighbor was out-of-town on a brief vacation. Was it luck or was it serendipity?

By Monday the basic court was completed, not the plastering or painting of the walls, but all the structural elements. It was time to execute the second part of the plan.

There were about a dozen homes in our small area, mostly young families with children. Knowing that there is strength in numbers, we went from house to house to invite adults and children to a mid-week cocktail/soda party. The purpose was to explain the "ugly structure" we had created in the neighborhood. Surprisingly, or perhaps not, everyone came with the exception of the angry neighbor across the way. Turns out, he was still out of town.

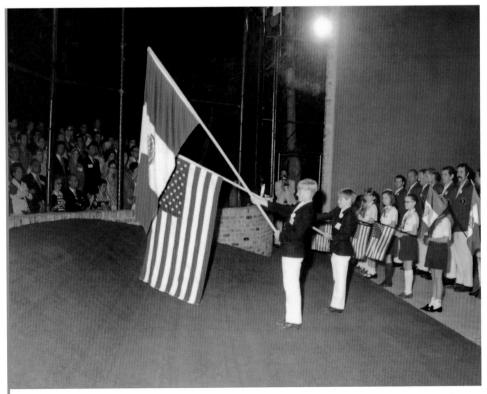

Inauguration ceremony at my fronton court in Houston, with many neighbors in attendance.

I was like the music man, explaining how everyone, especially the kids, could use the court. "A new game unique to all," is how I sold it. It was a gigantic success. The neighborhood supported the court 100 percent, in spite of some concern about the external finish on the walls. The interior was painted green, but the exterior was, quite frankly, an ugly gray. However, I had a prepared response: "No concern. We plan on using Chicago Common brick to cover all the external walls."

I really did not have that plan in mind, but since several homes in the neighborhood had that particular brick, it sounded like a smart move. That sealed the deal. They would support the project and resist any objection by the fellow across the way. Indeed, we were underway building the first fronton court for frontenis in the United States of America.

I had no misconception that someday I would be a world-class frontenis player, which indeed did not happen. However, the enjoyment the game provided family, students, fellow residents, hospital colleagues, and me was enough. After rounds on Saturday and Sunday afternoons, the gang migrated from the medical center to the fronton court. We played touch football, water basketball, and intense frontenis games, usually followed by hamburgers and hot dogs with plenty of beer. The neighborhood was peaceful, and the kids had their time on the court. There were no sightings of the ugly neighbor.

That would have been enough for me, but then Tommy Thompson, friend and author of the book *Hearts* I mentioned earlier, became part of the fronton gang. He engaged in some pretty aggressive competitions with the physicians. I didn't know it at the time, but Tommy was gathering information for a *Sports Illustrated* article he was preparing. On May 17, 1971, the following article appeared in the magazine:

A Doctor Tries a Transplant

It was hardly a minor operation, importing the slam-bang sport of frontenis from Mexico, but Heart Surgeon Ted Diethrich is so keen on the game he has built a lavish backyard court.   —*Thomas Thompson*

I never proofed or approved any of it, but the consequences reached farther than I realized. I learned that a group of racket sport enthusiasts had formed a United States Frontenis Sports Association. In fact, in 1968 the association fielded a team for the Mexican Olympics as a trial sport. Their results were disastrous, but that did not discourage them from persevering with the sport.

After leaving the operating room one morning, my secretary said there was a message to call home. I spoke with Gloria, and she relayed a conversation with a Mr. Richard Squires of the United States Frontenis Sports Association. He had become aware of my interest in the sport, as well as the fronton in my side yard. He wanted to meet me the next afternoon. I rearranged my schedule, and we met and hit a few balls. That was my tryout. Soon enough, I became a member of the United States Olympic Frontenis Team.

The major purpose of his visit was to enlist players to join the squad that would compete in the Vi Campeonato del Mundo de Pelota, held September 18– 27, 1971, in San Sebastian, Spain. I did not want to seem overly excited, but I could hardly contain myself. An Olympian playing in the World Games? It had to be a joke! But then again, the whole fronton endeavor had been somewhat unrealistic.

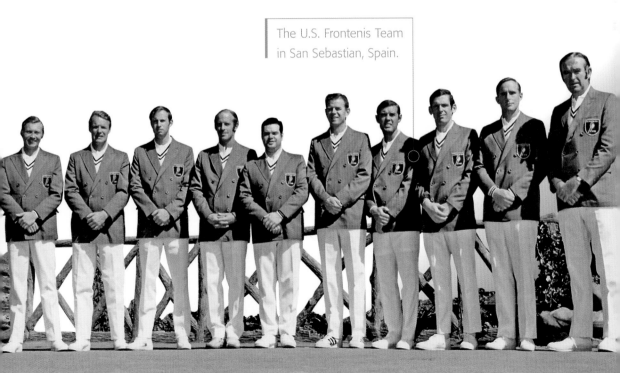

The U.S. Frontenis Team in San Sebastian, Spain.

Dick Squires sent me information regarding the games, and an official green jacket with the association logo on the pocket arrived soon after. The plan was for the team to assemble one week before the games for several days of practice. I made my airline reservations.

Upon arriving in San Sebastian, the U.S. team encountered a snafu. With all the teams coming to the games, there was a problem with too few courts for practice. Captain Dick set out to search for potential practice sites. About six hours later he called a team meeting—the problem had been solved. We would drive about thirty minutes outside the city to a convent. There would be no restrictions about scheduling practice time since only the U.S. team would be there. It seemed like an ideal solution.

Unfortunately, upon arrival we found the court had not been constructed for frontenis. It had a low ceiling and was not 100 feet long, but more like 150 feet long. There was little ventilation and definitely no air conditioning. Nevertheless we approached our practice with American enthusiasm.

About every hour or so we would take a much needed break and walk into the courtyard for some fresh air. We could see the nuns peering out of the upper floor windows, and when we waved they waved back. Some pretty-faced nuns soon appeared with soda and ice. They were so excited to be able to help solve our dehydration problem; they actually were a bit giddy.

The games were wonderful, and all of the Spanish pageantry was beautiful. Our team was terrible, with the exception of one dramatic event: a 30–20 upset against the French National team.

The second dramatic event of the tournament was the tragedy of a Basque nationalist who, drenched with gasoline, jumped from the balcony, and immolated himself on the fronton court in front of 3000 spectators, including Francisco Franco, dictator of Spain. He landed at the bench of the U.S. team, and a few of the ladies were slightly injured, particularly their hairdos.

I was very concerned about the possibility of severe burns, and indeed several spectators were taken to nearby hospitals. Fortunately, no one but the jumper was seriously injured. He was protesting Franco, who of course was quickly whisked from the building. It seemed the Basques were accustomed to such demonstrations. The match went on.

One evening upon returning to my hotel from the games, a message at the front desk requested that I call Dr. Hans Moore in Hamburg, Germany. I realized it must be the Dr. Moore from Philips that I interviewed in Houston to discuss angiography in the operating room.

We connected quickly, and he said he might have good news for me, and something to show me. Could I come to Hamburg to visit the University of Muenster before returning to the States? I could not pass on the opportunity and immediately changed my return air flight.

Two days later, Dr. Moore was escorting me into the emergency department in Muenster, Germany, and right before my eyes was the ceiling-mounted c-arm x-ray unit that I had envisioned months earlier. I knew it could not have been designed or constructed that rapidly. He explained that it was a "one off" unit they were using for emergency cases that involved arterial trauma. With his permission I examined every detail of the equipment; it was perfect for what I needed. Now came the big question, was it available?

"Not this one, but there is one other unfinished," he responded. If I had a checkbook in my pocket, I would have placed the order on the spot. As I returned to work in Houston, I anxiously waited for more details on the unit I had seen in Muenster.

Several weeks later, my secretary stepped in the office. "There is a Mr. Rudman who wishes to talk to you."

"Is he a patient?"

"He didn't divulge the reason for his call." I picked up the phone. "Dr. Diethrich speaking." Almost before I was done saying my name I heard, "This is M.B. Duke Rudman from Dallas, Texas. Are you the famous heart surgeon who loves to play fronton?"

I paused. "I'm not sure about the famous part, but you're correct about fronton." The caller then proceeded to explain the reasoning behind his phone call.

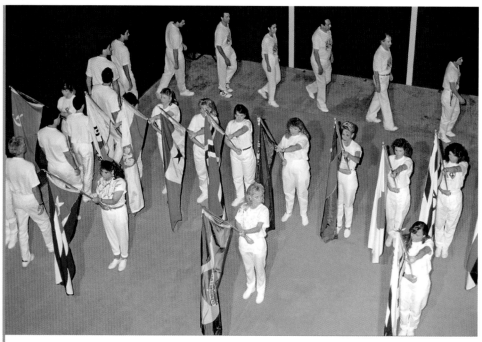

AHI staff participating in an International Frontenis ceremony at my home.

"I just finished construction on two new fronton courts on my ranch here in Dallas. When can you come over to play?"

"Well, I'll have to look at my calendar, maybe sometime in the next couple of months?" I replied.

"No, no, no. I mean now. I mean this weekend!" said the Duke.

That Saturday, a good friend and I flew to Mr. Rudman's Dallas home. He was an eccentric oilman, probably a billionaire as well, who had developed a shared obsession with the sport. We went to dinner at the country club, even bypassing dessert, and were soon on the courts, serving balls. It was freezing—a "blue norther," what they call a cold windstorm in Texas—had blown in, but it didn't matter. I had encountered another crazy guy who loved the sport. Now Texas had three frontons: my original in Houston and Duke's two.

In the following years, whenever I was in Dallas I would play with Duke's gang, and every February we went to Acapulco and were joined by several other players. These same folks, as well as players from all over the country, came to

Phoenix for tournaments when I built my first fronton court at the AHI facility in 1977.

It also became an AHI sport, where many of the staff would play early in the morning, at lunch, and in the evening. They also took an active part in the tournaments with flags, ceremonies, banners, and special posters with the names of the events. All of this furthered my endeavor to develop the AHI family no matter the activity.

The pride and core strength this developed within the team paid off enormously when there were cloudy skies in our future. This was exemplified to the maximum in my friendship with Duke Rudman. I learned friends are precious. I'm reminded of what a friend of mine once said, "If one has as many true friends that can be counted on one hand, he is a most fortunate person."

14

The Trump Card

Our work on the preservation chamber was a testimony to my concern about a future shortage of donor hearts—for all organs, actually. It occurred to me that there was a substantial "waste" of organs when one donor provides only a specific organ, such as a heart or a lung or maybe two kidneys. Why not develop a program where multiple organ transplants could be performed from just one donor?

While it seemed abundantly logical, it also bordered on a logistical nightmare. I posed this concept to my resident and now friend, John Liddicoat, and night after night, often very late, we would work in my home study developing the plan. The system needed to be practical, and the entire effort well documented.

What if a single phone call activated five operating rooms: one for the donor, two for the kidney recipients, one for a lung recipient, one for the heart recipient, and a room for audiovisual control? On a large drawing board we mapped out the plan.

The surgeons, support staff, and equipment required for each procedure were posted. When we were satisfied that every base was covered, it was time to expose the plan to one key person, but that person was not Dr. DeBakey. At that time, our team had not performed even one human heart transplant. The idea of simultaneous, multiple transplants might be a little bit for him to accept, but I would face that issue at the appropriate time.

The key person was Dana Estes, RN, then head of the Methodist operating rooms. We had become good friends, as she liked my efficiency and the respect I had gained with Dr. DeBakey. I ran the plan by her, not just once, but multiple times. She agreed it could be done; after all, there was an abundance of recipient patients, and the surgeons were eager to participate in the transplantation procedures.

With her blessing, I gradually talked to the key members who would participate. Everyone was geared up for a heart transplant, especially since Dr. Cooley had previously performed about a dozen at St. Luke's next door. Finding the donor was the next step.

While I explained my interest in music earlier, I never realized that it would eventually play a key role in a medical endeavor. The orchestration of music and medicine was constantly in sync in my life, so now, looking back, the fateful opportunity makes sense.

Dr. Grady Hallman, one of Dr. Cooley's associates, was an excellent trombone player. He assembled a group of doctors to form a band called the Heartbeats. I enjoyed playing the trumpet, but the lead was Dr. Warren Jacobs, an OB-GYN specialist. He had obviously kept his embouchure intact over the years. Dr. Cooley even played the bass fiddle. I'm not sure he ever made a sound on it, but he did look pretty legitimate acting the part in the back row.

The band became quite well known and we were asked to perform frequently, mostly for charitable occasions. Such was the case when the Heartbeats performed at the downtown St. Joseph's Hospital.

As we enjoyed refreshments after the performance, I was standing at the bar drinking a glass of wine next to one of the nurses. I introduced myself and explained I was on the transplant team from Methodist Hospital, and she replied that she worked in the intensive care unit. I jumped on the opportunity to explain that we were looking for organ donors, and if she became aware of one to please let me know. She seemed eager to help.

Two days later I received a call from St. Joe's. I was sure it was in reference to that conversation since I never went to that hospital. I immediately called John

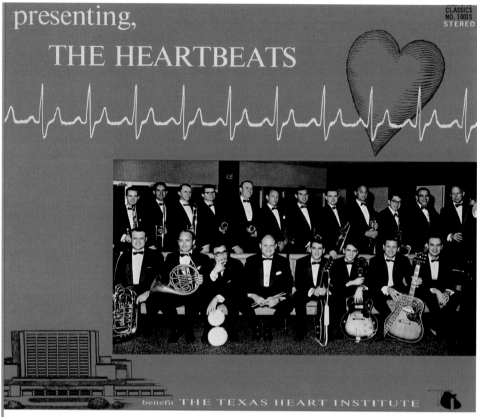

The cover of the Heartbeats Album.

with instructions to meet me at the office, and from there we drove to St. Joseph's Hospital in downtown Houston. Upon entering the ICU, I noted that there were no patients, just a draped-off area in one corner. Also, only one nurse was present, and it was not the pretty one from the wine reception. She also wasn't very friendly.

As I began to introduce myself, she raised her hand and pointed to the curtained off area. This was clearly a new experience for her as well. I examined the young lady on the respirator. I could not make a definitive judgment, but it was clear to me she was neurologically dead. I went back to the nurse and asked to see the husband.

"He is in jail," she replied. "There is suspicion that he shot her." John and I looked at each other. No husband, no release of the donor, no transplantation! Almost simultaneously we turned and left for the car, driving to the sheriff's office.

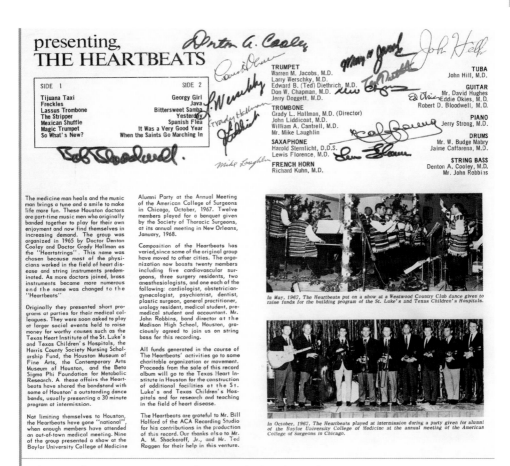

presenting, THE HEARTBEATS

SIDE 1	SIDE 2
Tijuana Taxi	Georgy Girl
Freckles	Java
Lassus Trombone	Bittersweet Samba
The Stripper	Yesterday
Mexican Shuffle	Spanish Flea
Magic Trumpet	It Was a Very Good Year
So What's New?	When the Saints Go Marching In

TRUMPET
Warren M. Jacobs, M.D.
Larry Werschky, M.D.
Edward B. (Ted) Diethrich, M.D.
Don W. Chapman, M.D.
Jerry Doggett, M.D.

TROMBONE
Grady L. Hallman, M.D. (Director)
John Liddicoat, M.D.
William A. Cantrell, M.D.
Mr. Mike Laughlin

SAXAPHONE
Harold Sternlicht, D.D.S.
Lewis Florence, M.D.

FRENCH HORN
Richard Kuhn, M.D.

TUBA
John Hill, M.D.

GUITAR
Mr. David Hughes
Eddie Okies, M.D.
Robert D. Bloodwell, M.D.

PIANO
Jerry Strong, M.D.

DRUMS
Mr. W. Budge Mabry
Jaime Caffarena, M.D.

STRING BASS
Denton A. Cooley, M.D.
Mr. John Robbins

The medicine man heals and the music man brings a tune and a smile to make life more fun. These Houston doctors are part-time music men who originally banded together to play for their own enjoyment and now find themselves in increasing demand. The group was organized in 1965 by Doctor Denton Cooley and Doctor Grady Hallman as the "Heartstrings". This name was chosen because most of the physicians worked in the field of heart disease and string instruments predominated. As more doctors joined, brass instruments became more numerous and the name was changed to the "Heartbeats"

Originally they presented short programs at parties for their medical colleagues. They were soon asked to play at larger social events held to raise money for worthy causes such as the Texas Heart Institute of the St. Luke's and Texas Children's Hospitals, the Harris County Society Nursing Scholarship Fund, the Houston Museum of Fine Arts, the Contemporary Arts Museum of Houston, and the Beta Sigma Phi Foundation for Metabolic Research. A. these affairs the Heartbeats have shared the bandstand with some of Houston's outstanding dance bands, usually presenting a 30 minute program at intermission.

Not limiting themselves to Houston, the Heartbeats have gone "national", when enough members have attended an out-of-town medical meeting. Nine of the group presented a show at the Baylor University College of Medicine

Alumni Party at the Annual Meeting of the American College of Surgeons in Chicago, October, 1967. Twelve members played for a banquet given by the Society of Thoracic Surgeons, at its annual meeting in New Orleans, January, 1968.

Composition of the Heartbeats has varied, since some of the original group have moved to other cities. The organization now boasts twenty members including five cardiovascular surgeons, three surgery residents, two anesthesiologists, and one each of the following: cardiologist, obstetrician-gynecologist, psychiatrist, dentist, plastic surgeon, general practitioner, urology resident, medical student, pre-medical student and accountant. Mr. John Robbins, band director at the Madison High School, Houston, graciously agreed to join us on string bass for this recording.

All funds generated in the course of The Heartbeats' activities go to some charitable organization or movement. Proceeds from the sale of this record album will go to the Texas Heart Institute in Houston for the construction of additional facilities at the St. Luke's and Texas Children's Hospitals and for research and teaching in the field of heart disease.

The Heartbeats are grateful to Mr. Bill Holford of the ACA Recording Studio for his contributions in the production of this record. Our thanks also to Mr. A. M. Shackeroff, Jr., and Mr. Ted Roggen for their help in this venture.

In May, 1967, The Heartbeats put on a show at a Westwood Country Club dance given to raise funds for the building program of the St. Luke's and Texas Children's Hospitals.

In October, 1967, The Heartbeats played at intermission during a party given for alumni of the Baylor University College of Medicine at the annual meeting of the American College of Surgeons in Chicago.

The Heartbeats were very popular at medical and social events .

Upon entering I was greeted by an overweight pleasant sheriff, who was obviously wondering what the two fellows in the long white coats and blue scrubs wanted at the county jail. I explained that we were from the transplant team at Methodist Hospital, and as we understood it, the husband of a possible donor was under his custody.

"Yes, we are holding Mr. Hernandez under suspicion of shooting his wife," he confirmed.

"May I go in and speak to him?" I requested. Without hesitation, the officer led me through the door leading to the husband's cell. Then without a word he opened the cell, let me in, and locked it behind him. *There must be some special power in these long white coats*, I thought. I told Mr. Hernandez that I was from the transplant team at Methodist Hospital. His wife had irreversible brain damage and would be appropriate as an organ donor. She could help save other patients if her organs were donated.

I wasn't quite sure he understood what I was explaining. I sat down beside him on the bunk. I put my arm on his shoulder, looked directly into his eyes and asked, "Mr. Hernandez did you shoot your wife?" He immediately broke down crying.

"No, no, I love her. I would never harm her. She has been very depressed lately and suddenly this morning took the revolver in the kitchen cabinet and shot herself in the head." He could hardly get the words from his mouth. I felt terrible. There I was, asking a man who loved his wife (and was being accused of killing her) for her organs. I gave him a big hug and confessed my sorrow, but still had to ask: "Would you sign the papers for the donation?"

He nodded yes. I rattled the cell door, and the sheriff approached and let me out. I turned to him and repeated my conversation with Mr. Hernandez. "Sheriff, this man did not kill his wife. He is deeply upset and wants to sign the consent for organ transplantation to help other desperate patients. Can you release him to me to go to St. Joseph's Hospital for the paperwork?"

"Dr. Diethrich, this sounds like a lifesaving situation. I'll sign the release." Within three minutes Mr. Hernandez was in the back seat of my car next to John, and I was speeding off to St. Joe's. Can you imagine that happening today? It was one of the most unbelievable experiences of my life—what a ride!

The scene in St. Joe's ICU had changed dramatically. The original nurse was nowhere in sight. Instead, there must have been twenty or thirty emotional family members gathered around the victim's bed. John produced the necessary papers, Mr. Hernandez signed, and another new nurse witnessed all of it to assure "compliance," a word we did not even have in those days.

It was time to initiate the plan we had worked on for months. The one phone call I had to make was to Dana at the Methodist operating room. "Dana, we have the donor, it's a go." She replied with an affirmative and hung up. While I was calling, John made ambulance arrangements for the transfer to Methodist.

When we arrived at Methodist there was already a buzz of activity in the air. I met with Dana, and she confirmed that the five operating rooms were being prepared—one donor, one lung, two kidneys, one heart, and an audiovisual area to coordinate the recording of this historic event that was about to unfold.

The donor had been placed in the rear of the ICU, and our EEG expert Peter Kellaway was standing by to begin his assessment. I made a quick sweep around the rooms, greeting the surgeons who would be participating. Everything was falling in line. There was only one missing link: I hadn't yet notified Dr. DeBakey, and we were already underway. Indeed, he had no idea of the multiorgan donation and transplantations.

I went back to the office and called him at home.

"Dr. DeBakey, I have wonderful news. We have a donor for Mr. Carroll, the heart patient who had been sent to me from Phoenix. Everything is progressing well. But there is even more good news. We are ready for the transplantation of the heart, a lung and two kidneys. All is underway."

His response was negative. "There is no way we can do all these procedures simultaneously. Forget the idea." He stopped talking. My heart sank.

Now what could I do? Everything was already well underway. I ran around to check each operating room—patients on the tables, surgeons scrubbing, and cameras rolling. Thirty minutes went by. I knew because I was checking my watch about every thirty seconds.

I could feel the beads of perspiration on my brow, and it reminded me of my first encounter with the OR Sister in Ann Arbor. It was back to the office to call Dr. DeBakey again.

"Everything is working perfectly. Please come over right away," I repeated.

"Ted, we don't have enough blood for all these procedures." He hung the phone up again. That made me nervous, so I called the blood bank to verify it wasn't a problem; they had plenty on reserve. Another twenty minutes passed before I called him again. This time I was desperate.

"Dr. DeBakey, please come to the hospital right away. We have five operations going and you need to be here." The line went dead.

Ten minutes later I heard his footsteps coming down the long corridor. He stopped and looked at me. "Where is the donor?" I quickly led him to the ICU to see Peter and note the EEG, and purposely stood several feet away.

After only a brief time (although it seemed like hours to me) he yanked the curtain open and stormed out of the cubicle, racing back toward his office. I was half a pace behind. My mind was swirling. *What had I done?* My entire surgical career was about to be destroyed. In my enthusiasm for this endeavor, I had stepped over the boundary.

We were about to pass through the vacant x-ray department, and I knew if I didn't act quickly it was curtains down. I paused and nudged him by the elbow into the semi-dark x-ray room. It was cold, but I was hot with perspiration. Even my hands were shaking. I had no plan, but then the words came strong and clear from my mouth.

"Dr. DeBakey, do you think that Dr. Cooley would ever pass up an opportunity like this?" He paused in his reflection, as I stood rigid as a statue.

"Ted, you're right. Proceed!"

I had played the Trump Card in desperation.

All of the procedures went well, including the procurement of both corneas. The Fonden-Brown Building had just been opened with its connecting bridge to Methodist Hospital. Several of the ICUs there were prepared for transplantation patients but had not yet received any before the multiple-organ transplantation.

The plan was to open one cardiac ICU to receive Bill Carroll, the heart transplant recipient. Upon completion of the heart operation, I accompanied other members of the team to the new unit across the bridge.

The first priority was to connect the respirator to the electrical outlet, so the anesthesiologist would not have to continue the respirations manually. I plugged the respirator into the wall socket—but it did not turn on. I tried the other two outlets several times, and it was clear they were non-functional, whether it was a failing plug, circuit breaker issue, or some other mechanical electrical malfunction. I spoke to the head nurse and ordered an extension cord from engineering. Ten minutes later it arrived, we connected it to a wall outlet in the next room, and the respirator began to function immediately.

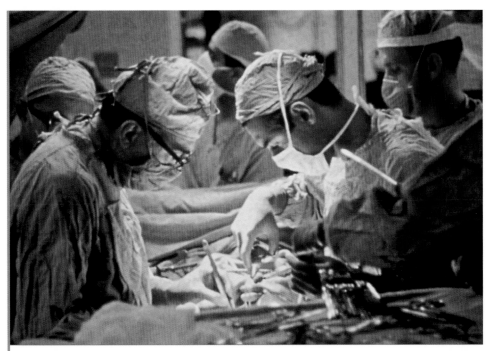

Dr. DeBakey assisting me with the heart transplant in the first multiple organ transplantation procedure. Dr. Liddicoat, co-planner of the event, is standing behind me.

Who would believe that such an historic operation could be derailed by a simple electrical wall socket, but then put back on track with the aid of an extension cord?

An hour later, Bill Carroll was awake.

Around nine in the morning it was announced that there was a press conference in the cafeteria at 11 a.m., scheduled by Dr. DeBakey and Ted Bowen, the hospital CEO. The room was packed and the press were everywhere with cameras and note pads. Mr. Bowen began with the usual greeting and announcement of the historic operation. He did not mention it was performed just a few hundred feet down the tunnel from Dr. Cooley's operating theater.

Dr. DeBakey followed with a flowing speech about the significance of the procedure. Many more transplants could be performed, costs would be reduced, and lives saved. He was in good form, giving details and answering questions from the press like the proud father of a first-born son. It ended with a standing ovation from the crowded audience.

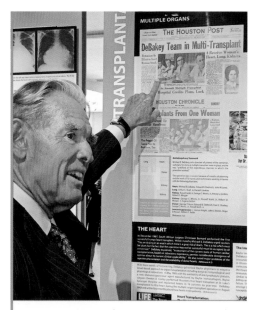

I am pointing to the *Houston Post* article in the DeBakey library on the multiple organ transplant during a recess in the DeBakey Society meeting in Houston, Texas.

John and I sat there, quietly reflecting on the past months of preparation and the final hours of executing the quadruple operation. It had all been successful, despite what seemed like insurmountable obstacles, from the county jail scene to Dr. DeBakey's strong initial resistance.

We shook hands, both exhausted. We knew what we had achieved. Even a poor electrical plug could not stop us from the ultimate goal.

Dr. DeBakey had not offered one word of appreciation or acknowledgment regarding our orchestration of the symphonic quality performance. It was not the lack of recognition that affected me; rather, it was the realization that this was Dr. DeBakey's empire, and he would reign over it for years as its king. There was no future pathway for a prince in his vision. I could accept that, but I would have to look for my own kingdom.

I called home a little later and spoke to Gloria, telling her the story in an abbreviated version. I ended the conversation saying, "Gloria, we are going to leave Houston. I am not sure when, but I cannot stay here." She was shocked but did not argue. She knew we would talk later.

There were no charges brought against Mr. Hernandez. I sensed there was extreme passion for the husband who had to bury his organ-less wife.

A few months ago, in May 2014, I was at the Michael E. DeBakey Department of Surgery Alumni Symposium and visited the DeBakey library. One of the exhibitions that caught my attention was the multiorgan transplant.

There it was, DeBakey, reigning over his kingdom. I knew I had made the right decision.

15

"Heart" Felt Dreams

In late August 1969, months after the multiorgan transplant, it was time to have a conversation with Dr. DeBakey about my future interests in research, education, and clinical care. He actually had made appointments for me with three university programs outside of Texas that were seeking someone to establish a cardiovascular unit similar to the one in Houston.

Each time I returned, I reported the environment would not be conducive because there was too much competition between departmental chairmen. They were operating in the typical silo format. Henry Ford Hospital, the Lahey Clinic in Boston, and several large cardiovascular practice groups had also contacted me. None of these seemed to fit my dream for the future. In my head, I began to mold a plan into shape. So I summoned my courage.

I had mentally rehearsed for the twelfth time what I would say and asked Dr. DeBakey for a private audience. I spoke quickly and enthusiastically, looking directly into his magnified eyes behind the thick glasses. I told him I would be resigning. I had been privately working on a dream to build my own heart institute, and now it was far enough along to be assured.

"I am going to Phoenix, Arizona," I told him. I had found backers to build a $3 million addition to an existing Catholic hospital, and I planned on forming my own team of cardiologists, nurses, pump technicians, and staff. There might be affiliations with the University of Arizona Medical School.

Dr. DeBakey did not attempt to dissuade me, even though I was a valuable member of his team. If successful, the Arizona Heart Institute would serve the Southwest, a portion of the country that sent hundreds of patients to Houston. "Keep me informed," was all he said.

The following is my description of the plan as told to Tommy Thompson from a section of *Hearts*:

* With the long-kept-quiet cat finally out of the bag, I spoke with excitement as I began recruiting. "It's going to be FAN-TAS-TIC," I fairly cried. "Suppose a doctor calls up and says, "I've got a 45-year-old man who's just had an acute coronary, what can you do for him?" Well, the Arizona Heart Institute will have on hand a 24-hour-a-day ambulance with a doctor inside. They go out, bring this man in, not to the emergency room of a hospital, but to an area in our Institute that is equipped for everything from minor IV support to coronary catheterization to immediate bypass surgery. Nobody has this concept yet. This is the Outer Space Medicine of the future. We can pick up patients by helicopter from 200 miles around. We'll have our own jet, too. When somebody calls in sick from Chicago, what can we do for him? We can do many things for him! We can send our jet out to get him and perhaps save his life. The philosophy of so many doctors is 20 years back—100 years back. They give a heart-attack victim an ECG, put him to bed, and start him on exercise. I'm not at all sure that you shouldn't start exploring vessels right away, do cardiac catheterization immediately upon his arrival at the hospital. We have surgical methods now to immediately revascularize the heart, to immediately restore a new blood supply. If you look at statistics of coronary death rate of people admitted to hospitals who have low blood pressure on arrival, 75% of them never leave the hospital. This doesn't even take into consideration the 50% who never even arrive.

These may seem like wild, far-out ideas, but these are things I could never develop in Houston. There's no way for me to form my own team. I can't sit around another five or ten years until Dr. DeBakey retires. When he leaves, there's going to be the maddest scramble for power you have ever seen. We're going to start clean in Arizona.

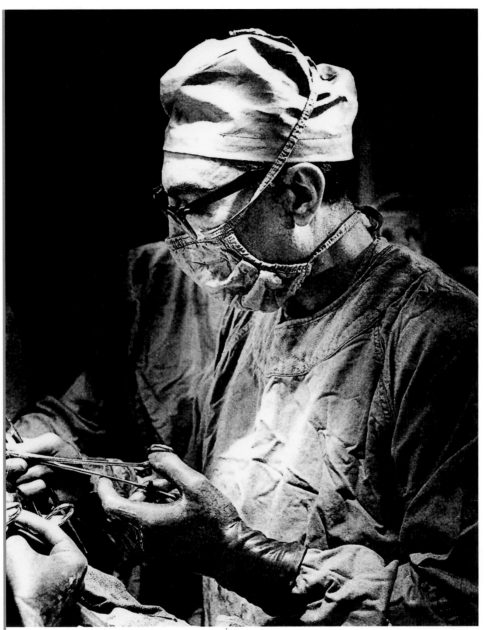

To Ted Dittrich –
with high esteem for
his surgical capabilities
and his academic endeavors
and with warm friendship

Michael E DeBakey

Michael E. DeBakey, MD, presented me with this photo on my departure from Houston.

I'm going to have only people who can get excited. People that you can't excite, I'm through with. I have to have people beside me that you can light a bomb under and they're in orbit, seven days a week. I want a handful of people with me who can change the world of heart care.

Thinking back, I remembered a morning when Dr. Cooley motioned for me to come to his office above the operating room at St. Luke's Hospital. He proudly showed me a prototype of the Texas Heart Institute logo he was intending to use for his dream of a new institute.

It was quite obviously not an open discussion for many, since the DeBakey team was tunneled only a short distance away. Peering at the logo, the gears in my mind started turning, and I realized he was actually showing me what I might create a thousand miles to the west one day. It was just far too early for me to be considering logos.

The dream was clear, but the plan of execution uncertain. It wasn't like I had my own Houston team that could move half way across the country to try a potentially risky adventure. A cardiologist was essential, especially one highly skilled in catheterization. So I only asked one: the doctor called "Super Sam the Cath Man." In most people's opinion, he was number one on Dr. DeBakey's team.

I told him of my plan, invited him to join me, and waited four long days without any reply. Suddenly, he appeared in my office, came over to my desk, shook my hand, and said, "We are coming with you." The "we" referred to his wonderful wife, Aimee Ann.

I was ecstatic. The first brick had been laid in the new Arizona Heart Institute, and it was a special one. Several other key positions would need to be filled, including an

Dr. Sam Kinard, also known as Super Sam the Cath Man.

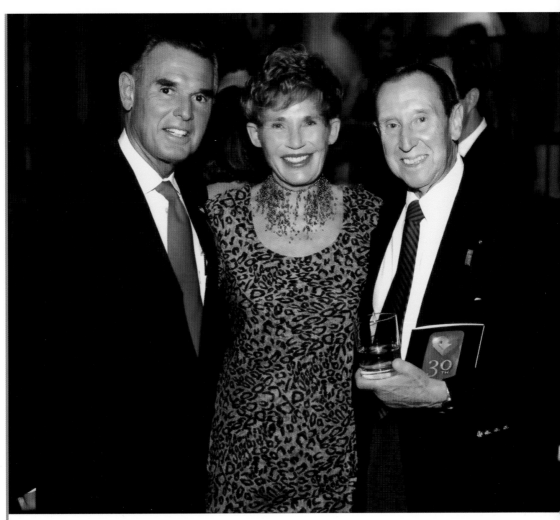

Drs. Joe and Carolyn Gerster. Joe called me when he read the announcement about the Arizona Heart Institute being established in Phoenix. Until that time, both cardiologists referred their heart surgery patients to Denton Cooley in Houston. They later became the most loyal supporters of the AHI program; my friend Joe died June 21, 2015.

audiovisual expert. That may seem strange, but AV was not only a hobby—it was a fundamental component of my vision for the Institute.

The first paid employee was a cinematographer. The second, an operating room nurse from Methodist Hospital named Mildred Coram, who had great organizational skills. She soon left for Phoenix to become the Institute Project Director at St. Joseph's Hospital and Medical Center, founded by the Sisters of Mercy.

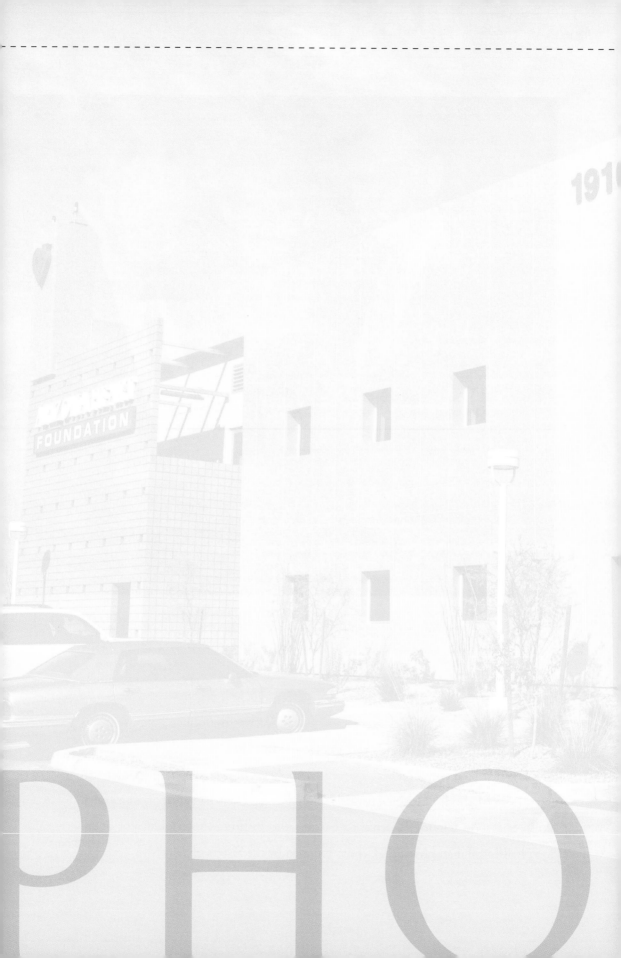

PHOENIX

16

Life in Phoenix,
A Big Dose of Reality

I arrived in Phoenix in 1971 after several encouraging conversations with two cardiology brothers who had recruited me to move to the Valley to build a cardiovascular surgical program at St. Joseph's Hospital and Medical Center. That sounded good, but I had a much more comprehensive vision for a different kind of project all together. I wanted to create a center dedicated to the detection, treatment, and prevention of heart disease, not just specific to the Southwest but as a resource for the entire world. My whole life reflects a belief in education—of young students, nurses, fellows, residents, and of course, the general population. (A priority for me has always been to "stamp out heart disease," a goal that was highly endorsed by the Arizona Heart Foundation Board of Directors, most especially our chairman, Jess Nicks, father of the famous singer Stevie Nicks.)

In order to successfully make a dent in these goals, the public needed to be educated about the risk factors for cardiovascular

Jess Nicks, former AHF Board Chairman, with his daughter, singer and performer Stevie Nicks, before a benefit concert for the Arizona Heart Foundation.

disease, as well as the latest diagnostic tools to detect this disease and the various approaches to treat it. My vision for the Institute was that with new techniques and advanced teaching, coupled with public and professional education, our team would be able to change the world of heart care as it was known at that time.

The reality of starting my "private practice" in Phoenix in 1971 was to be challenging in so many ways, some unimaginable to me at the time. I had always been associated with schools or universities emphasizing academics. Some had provisions for limited private practice, but most were salaried positions. Overall, I was insulated by the academic institutions' infrastructure and dominance. That statement might seem obvious, since most of the stories told up to now could not have occurred without such protection. I was constantly on the cutting edge, barely avoiding a self-inflicted injury.

St. Joseph's Hospital, the home of the new Arizona Heart Institute (AHI), did not provide a security blanket for its new cardiovascular center, nor did I think that it was important when establishing the program. I had not yet, however, encountered my first rattlesnake.

Physicians entering the medical community in Phoenix were asked to become a member of the Maricopa County Medical Society. I was eager to join, and as part of the application process, I was interviewed by the society's ethics committee chairman, William Helm, a neurosurgeon. Dr. Helm conducted a very friendly interview, right up until he mentioned the publicity about the experimental multi-organ transplantation when I was in Houston. I did not think much about it until he read a passage from the ethics committee rules regarding the protocol of conduct for physicians and their relationship with the press and the public. It was highly restrictive.

My response was that one of my missions was to educate the public about heart disease and its prevention. Why would we build a program like AHI and not utilize it to inform the public what they needed to know relative to preventing heart and blood vessel disease? I made it clear that I intended to have public meetings and deal with the media freely.

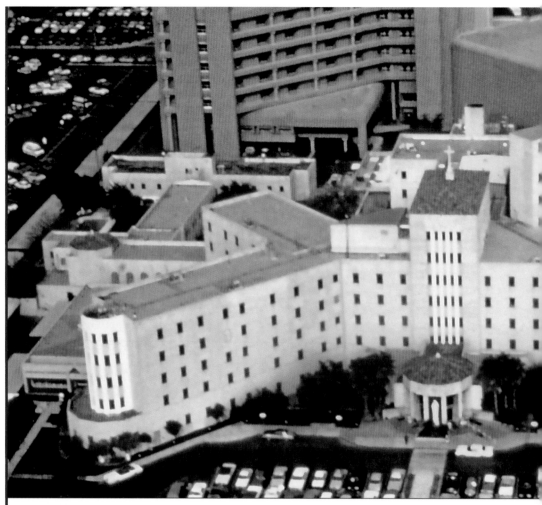

The original St. Joseph's Hospital and Medical Center in the early 1970s. The Arizona Heart Institute was located in the right wing of the hospital near Barrow Neurological Institute.

I received a firm response that such activity would be strictly forbidden. It was instantly clear that this board, and for that matter the physician community at large, had no appreciation of my plans regarding public relations for the AHI. I was not only in rattlesnake country, but surrounded by a bunch of highly conservative cowboy doctors. They had little or no interest in a broad-based plan to address cardiovascular disease by going directly to where that culprit attacked: the public. My plan was extensive and well sculptured, but it indeed had created a negative local effect, just like the transplantation event so successfully executed earlier in

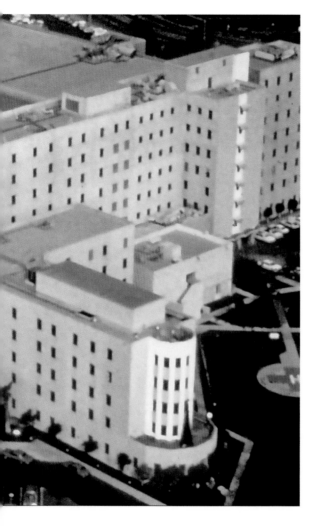

Houston. I stood up, excused myself, and asked that my application be withdrawn. First rattlesnake encounter lost, at least for the present.

The concept of a "closed staff" was another important difference between the public or private hospital and the academic centers. In the latter only faculty members had privileges to practice, whereas in the former, any physicians with qualifications could operate. In talking to Dr. DeBakey about my plans, he firmly believed I should insist on a closed staff. He felt that was the only way to assure the highest quality of care and internal peer review. I understood his position, as I was raised in this system and experienced it at the Henry Ford Hospital in Detroit. The chief executive nun of St. Joseph's, Sister Mary DePaul Oberti, agreed and a closed staff was incorporated into my contract.

To my amazement, on the day the Institute opening was announced, Sister Mary stood before the press and extolled that AHI would have an open staff where all qualified doctors could practice. I immediately challenged her, but her response was simply that "it would be better for the community."

It was clear that I was going to have a battle regarding the closed staff issue, not only with the surgeons but also the anesthesiologists who supported that policy. They would go from hospital-to-hospital: put the patient to sleep, wake the patient up, and hop in the car to the next operating room, sometimes to several within

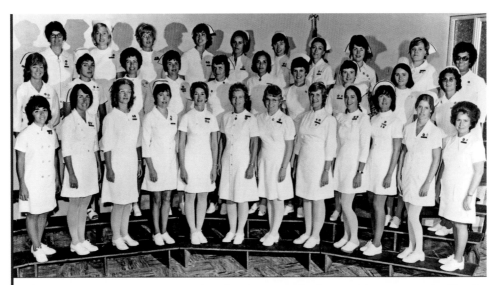

It became necessary to create an educational program for the special nurses required for the cardiovascular program. This is the first graduating class in 1972, a year after we began the Arizona Heart Institute. (Do you see any resemblance to Nina Amanda Kilgore, RN?)

one day. This was completely unacceptable to me, and I soon recognized that this was the same exact pattern for some of the surgeons. I solved the anesthesia issue; within a month after multiple arguments, I had my own anesthesiology team. The surgeons were another story.

When I decided to leave Baylor and build the AHI, I felt totally prepared to meet and overcome any obstacle. After all, I had survived the ultimate test of Dr. DeBakey. I thought nothing could be worse than that. Looking back now, it's hard to see how I could have been so naïve not to appreciate the early warning signs. Yes, the Medical Society's ethics committee bringing up the publicity in Houston was a red flag. And while the nun's announcement that the Institute would be open staff was critical, I thought we would overcome that with sheer volume. Soon, the very cardiologists who had campaigned for me to come to Phoenix turned against me when they did not get a coveted ECG contract they expected from the leverage of my position as AHI Director. Little did I know the breadth of their influence, the depth of their antagonism, or that I was about to inadvertently fan their smoldering resentment.

17

LIFE at AHI

One day in 1972 when the Institute at St. Joe's Hospital had been open about a year, a writer from *LIFE* magazine contacted me. They had just done a special presentation on the brain, and the description of technique and science was very impressive. They proposed doing a similar article on the heart and the work we were doing at the Institute. After several conversations I eventually felt comfortable with their proposal. In fact, I thought it would be a great way for the public to gain the knowledge they needed in order to take better care of themselves, thus preventing heart attacks (still our number one killer today).

The lead writer, Rick Gore, and his cameraman were in Phoenix for more than a week to gather research and observe our work. During this time I went about my practice as usual. Innocently, I did not feel I had to restrict them, unless it came to patient confidentiality. They followed me around, we had meals together, and I spoke to them freely about what they were observing. During that week we also had our usual basketball game that included fellows and staff. It was part of our "fitness" initiative. On the weekend I took them water-skiing with my son at Canyon Lake. In short, they were living a typical week in my life's schedule.

Not too long after their departure, the writer called and asked a few technical questions. He also said there was a lot of excitement at *LIFE* about the article, and it might even be front cover material.

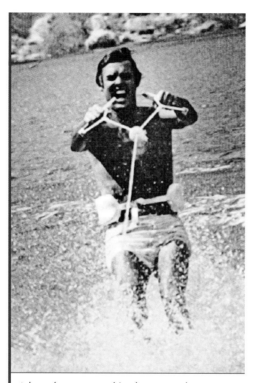

I loved to water-ski whenever there was a break in the schedule. My staff enjoyed the outings on Canyon Lake as well.

LIFE never sent us an advance copy; therefore, I had no opportunity to edit the article in any way. Frankly, I anticipated an article very much like the brain story that had convinced me to do the project in the first place. I will never forget the moment I first saw the article on October 13, 1972. Splashed across the cover (They didn't lie; it was on the cover.) read, "The daring heart surgeon they call Ted Terrific." My first thought was, *where did that come from?* Then I opened the pages to see Marie Alexander, our perfusionist, in a long lab coat with "Ted Terrific" imprinted on the back. It was a birthday party with my staff and friends present, and the "Ted Terrific" was an expression of respect and admiration, (maybe even love) for me as the team leader. Either way, it was all in fun for the spirit of a birthday party captured forever in print by *LIFE* magazine. To this day I wonder why the short title above Ted Terrific was "Shake Up in the FBI."

The *LIFE* article was more focused on depicting a surgeon on a fast track of fast cars, fast water skiing, fast basketball games, and playing fast frontenis. It was nothing like I had expected or hoped it would look like. Needless to say, this infuriated my colleagues at St. Joseph's Hospital, and soon I found this went even beyond the confines of Phoenix. Before the *LIFE* article, I only had to deal with small battles. This publication was a declaration of worldwide war against Ted Diethrich.

Interestingly, soon after the publication, I received an unsolicited letter from the writer of the *LIFE* article.

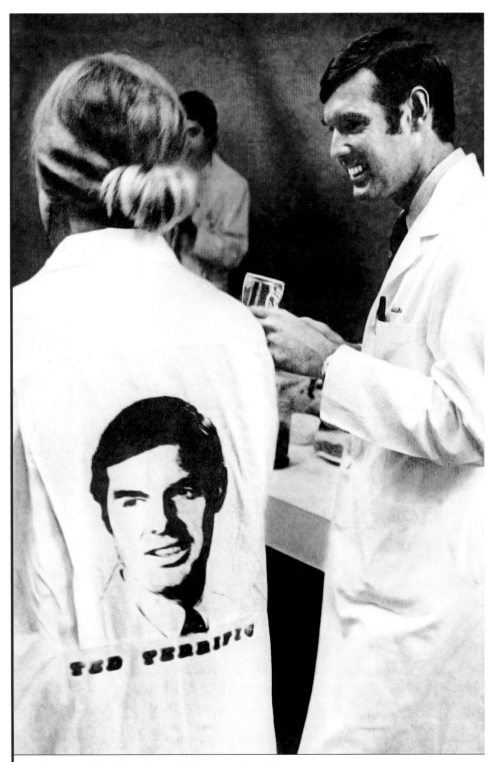

The innocent birthday photo which created a nightmare.

TIME & LIFE BUILDING
ROCKEFELLER CENTER
NEW YORK 10020
JUDSON 6-1212

October 30, 1972

Dr. Edward B. Diethrich
Arizona Heart Institute
350 West Thomas Road
Phoenix, Arizona 85013

Dear Dr. Diethrich:

I have heard through the medical grapevine that you are suffering
an intense backlash from the story we did on you in our October 13
issue. I am most sorry that the approach our staff in New York decided
to take has brought you embarrassment and a threat to your professional
standing. I want to make a statement regarding the preparation of that
article:

I had been looking for some time for a story that would focus on
the controversy surrounding the vein bypass technique, a controversy
that certainly was much in the news media this year. Also, the science
department of LIFE had for some time -- even before he left Houston--
been interested in doing a story on Dr. Edward Diethrich. He combined
the professional credentials with a personality that seemed to me to
epitomize the cardiac surgeon. His work encompassed the latest in heart
technology as well as the current bypass debate. Examining the person-
alities of doctors, particularly those in such vital areas as heart
surgery, is, I believe, as legitimate a function of journalism as discussing our politicians. Dr. Diethrich, I most strongly stress, did not
seek out the kind of publicity the article apparently has brought. What
may sound to some in the article like him pushing the bypass approach
is Ted Diethrich's natural enthusiasm for what he does.

We approached Dr. Diethrich about doing a story when we heard that
the Arizona Heart Institute was in full operation. We intended to
focus on the science involved primarily. Obviously a larger and richer
story evolved after we arrived in Phoenix and observed the refreshing
zeal of the man and the AHI staff. Our presentation was the way I, our
photographer Mike Mauney and eventually our editors in New York viewed
Diethrich and the institute. At first even I had no idea how strongly
the finished story would focus on Dr. Diethrich personally. And Dr.
Diethrich did not know it until the magazine hit the newsstands. He
resisted the popularization while we were in Phoenix. He asked us not
to use the nickname "Ted Terrific" or the photograph with the girl

dressed in the silkscreened surgical gown. I did not respect his request because it was my judgement that since the name and the picture
arose spontaneously from the staff — and because they so accurately
described the layman's impression of the man —-they were appropriate to
the story. Dr. Diethrich made very strenuous efforts to expose us to
the science and technology involved in his operations. He had an
assistant with us full time to make sure our technical questions were
answered. I fully intended to report on the subtleties involved in
the technology but did not get sufficient text space in the end to do
so. He explained fully his reliance on St. Joseph's Hospital for
support. Since I was working with minimal text space, I could only
mention the hospital once.

   Dr. Diethrich was open enough to permit us to see both his successes
and failures. He reluctantly permitted us to photograph him off-hours,
at home and enjoying sports after we told him we needed to humanize the article. The informal pictures obviously turned out to be journalistically
some of the most outstanding. These are the facts. We portrayed
Dr. Diethrich and the institute as we saw him. I believe our portrait was
accurate and appropriate. I think it would be most unfortunate if this
remarkable and talented man had to suffer professionally from our decisions and his own forthrightness and openness in dealing with the public.
If the story offended some people and some sensitivities, I am sorry.

                                        Most cordially,

                                        Rick Gore

Wherever I went in the United States, Europe, or South America, it was all the same. With each introduction before I spoke, a photo of the *LIFE* magazine cover would appear on the screen, and I was introduced as Ted Terrific.

While I might make an attempt to joke about it, I finally recognized that many in the audience did not approve. It was clearly against tradition. Rick Gore's reference in his letter to me regarding "suffering an intense backlash from the *LIFE* story" was clearly a gross understatement. I could have survived those occasions, but when I was censored by the American College of Surgeons and required to make a public apology before their board, it was heart breaking. Even worse than that punishment was the fact I could not publish a scientific article or make a presentation in any way associated with the College. Can you imagine what a blow this was to me? I am attempting to build a cardiovascular program in Phoenix with all the finest

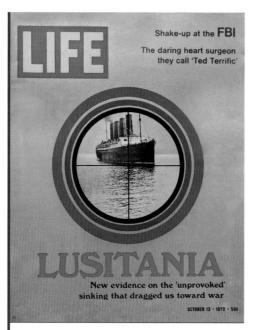

Shake-up at the **FBI**

The daring heart surgeon
they call 'Ted Terrific'

LUSITANIA

New evidence on the 'unprovoked'
sinking that dragged us toward war

OCTOBER 13 · 1972 · 50¢

I always wondered why they had an article titled, "Shake up at the FBI" right above the name of my article.

characteristics of research, education, and clinical care, and suddenly I found my hands tied behind my back.

When I left the disciplinary meeting of the American College of Surgeons that day in Chicago, I turned out of the front door of the building and walked miles down Michigan Avenue, not able to control my emotions. How could I have made such an error in judgment? This was truly a wakeup call! *LIFE* had actually shown me how cruel people can be. When challenged out of their comfort zone, they coil and prepare to strike, just like the desert rattlesnake.

An interesting side bar to this *LIFE* magazine article was brought to my attention in reading Dr. Cooley's book *100,000 Hearts*. He notes that Texas Heart's reputation continued to grow and brought more attention to Houston as a cardiovascular center. He mentions in his book:

> *However, in one instance we didn't get the attention we thought we deserved. In 1972, THI had its 10,000 open-heart case, a number that included about 1,900 coronary bypasses. Not only was this number of overall cases huge, but our survival rate of 98 percent was also amazing for the time. The story was offered to the medical editor of* LIFE *magazine, who said that another story about heart surgery was already scheduled, so a second one wasn't needed. "Call us back if you do something exciting" he said. As we later found out, the article that bumped our story from* LIFE *was about my trainee Ted Diethrich and his recent founding of the Arizona Heart Institute.*

18

The Medical Mafia

I was never going to include this part of my story in this book, but after intense urging from friends, I thought I would try to relate this particularly dark time in my life, a really bad ride.

I spoke earlier about our first hurdle when AHI opened, with the community directly challenging the "closed staff" concept. It wasn't long before we encountered another obstacle related to our research activities, one that would have repercussions far and wide.

I had a conversation with Bill Gore, the founder of W.L. Gore & Associates in Flagstaff, Arizona, about developing a graft for use as an artificial vessel. Gore had brought me a piece of tubing, which was actually a material for insulation, and asked if I thought it would be useful in my vascular work. I told him we could do some animal work and see the results.

I had recently hired an associate surgeon to work at AHI. We had research space at Arizona State University, so I assigned the project to him. He encouraged me to sign on one of his fellow trainees from an east coast university. Later without my knowledge, this associate joined a Gore employee and others to set up a research team and formed another company to do the exact same graft development, all in total secrecy. Amidst all of the lies and the cover-ups, basically I believed they had stolen Gore's design and feigned ignorance. This led perhaps to the longest lawsuit in medical industry history, sixteen years, between Gore and Impra, the new company with whom my own staff members were working. Gore eventually lost the lawsuit, and interestingly enough I was never asked for, nor did I ever give, a deposition. This story in itself deserves its own book.

Subsequently, we had to relieve this surgeon from any research responsibilities for the Institute, eventually discharging him altogether. This only led to further trouble with the closed staff issue. A black cloud was beginning to form over our heads, but I didn't know the deluge that was coming until a retired physician from the Mayo Clinic in Rochester, Minnesota, stopped by my office. It was 1972 before the "Ted Terrific" article hit the press. I had first met the doctor when I visited Mayo's before beginning the Arizona Heart Institute; he was now living in Sun City, Arizona. As he sat down for a chat, he showed me a book he was carrying. It was about the Mayo brothers' beginning their clinic. He had marked a certain section for my special attention.

"This will give you some idea of how the brothers struggled against the established medical community," he told me as he got up to leave. Then he stopped and turned to shake my hand.

"Ted, last evening I went to a meeting where there were twenty or thirty doctors. The only purpose of that meeting was to figure out how they were going to ruin your practice and force you to leave town. They talked about trumping up malpractice cases, filing complaints to the State Board of Medical Examiners, and creating negative publicity about you personally and the practice at the Institute. It reminded me of the stories of the Ku Klux Klan. I wish I could tell you their names, but I can't. I can tell you, however, that they are your surgical competitors." He pointed to the book again. "Read it and take heed. Good luck."

Stunned, I read the book he gave me and began to compare it to my current situation. It was then I realized what I was dealing with the "Medical Mafia." It's true what they say. If you think you have a problem with them, you do. If you don't think you have a problem with them, but they think you do, well, then you do.

These physicians (alluded to by the Mayo doctor) were meeting secretly at country club lunches, golf outings, and at each other's homes to discuss and invent stories about my medical practice, quality of work, and publicity. In the early '70s, physicians were not in the media to any extent; as the medical society interview made clear, it was considered unethical. However, I did not search for these public relations opportunities; they came naturally as we told the story of our work. The *LIFE* magazine article was a perfect example. Nevertheless, this type of media frenzy infuriated the local physicians. Now more than ever they hated me, hated my work, hated my insistence on public education, hated my acceptance of the sickest patients who would die if not operated on, and most of all hated my ability to succeed. They were insanely jealous.

Physicians and surgeons boycotted referrals and began to freeze me out to every extent possible. These physicians wanted me to go back to Houston (or any place but Phoenix) with my tail between my legs. More false stories began to circulate.

They wanted to review all of my cases to look for some reason to indict me. It was clear to me that I was the outsider in this so-called friendly process, later to be categorized and known as "peer review." They met with hospital lawyers who worked endlessly to gather what they thought were the facts about many botched cases, unnecessary surgeries, and patients who died. Ad hoc committees were formed with no request from me to answer the charges, creating more investigations. On top of everything, this witch hunt was confidential. I could not even obtain the specific list of charges or the names of my accusers. Physicians removed their children from the same school my children attended. Even my family became outcasts. I was removed as Medical Director of the Institute and some of my surgical privileges were suspended. Inside of fifteen months, I was sued eight times for malpractice all by the same attorney, a friend of my conspirators. This was serious.

It became clear to me that the "Medical Mafia" was not just a local association. My inability to join the Maricopa County Medical Society precluded my membership in the American Medical Association. As part of a restriction on operative privileges, I was required to perform five mitral valve cases under preoperative clearance. It got to the point where the Arizona Board of Medical Examiners was even considering revocation of my license.

It was a nightmare for someone who really did not understand the "organized hatred." It's endless, it's real, and it doesn't go away. Every corner you turn, you run into another problem you don't know how to solve, especially when you can't see the specific allegations against you. How could I possibly respond? I had few weapons to fire. A very good friend and AHI board member, Tom Chauncey, who headed the local CBS station, would call me every morning after reading the

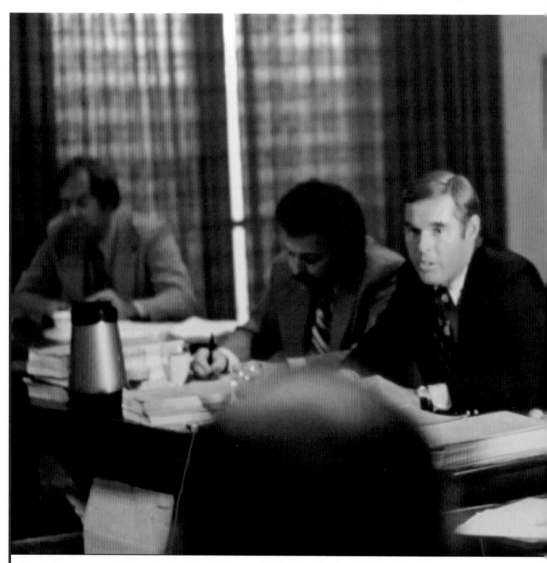

My defense team deliberating before the State Board of Medical Examiners. Their arguments were ultimately overwhelmingly successful. The allegations were a total sham. Phil Hirschkop is to my right and Ed Hendricks is to my left.

headlines. We had the same very brief conversation. "Keep your mouth shut!" he would recommend. And I listened.

Early one Sunday morning, I was still sleeping when the phone rang. I answered, thinking it would be the hospital.

"Morning Ted, Duke here. I'm hearing you are in big trouble out there with no good help. I want you to call this number. It is Phillip Hirschkop in Washington.

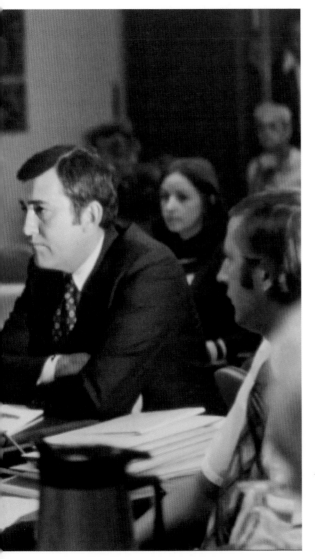

He is the famous attorney defending the Hunt brothers in the Texas lawsuit involving their late father's estate. You need his help. I have alerted him to expect your call."

I thanked Duke, and we hung up. It would come to pass that this call from a precious friend saved my medical career.

The following Monday evening I was sitting in a hotel lounge in St. Louis, waiting to speak with Phillip Hirschkop. He was traveling there to see another client. I waited very patiently for three hours until he finally appeared and introduced himself. I began to tell my story. Several hours later he stood, looked me right in the eye, and said, "You are being screwed over by a bunch of your own profession. Duke is right. You do need help. I'm going to take your case on and whip those bastards."

That was the beginning of hope. I had been in the ring and was on the verge of being knocked out. I re-read the Mayo brothers' marked chapter on the way back home. I was beginning to understand what they had gone through to achieve success. I could not wait for Phil to arrive in Phoenix and tell me his plan, which began with exposing the physicians who were hiding in the wings.

Hirschkop filed a $100 million lawsuit against nine physicians, the hospital, and several medical associations, charging them with antitrust violations, conspiracy, and restraint of trade. What I failed to realize was that when a lawsuit is filed, it immediately opens the potential to take depositions under oath. For the first time, the truth would finally come out. The scenario was repeated with each deposition. The whole charade was a giant orchestration of smoke and mirrors. Phil and his team began to fracture those mirrors and the faces behind them. The accusers had to begin to divulge their sources. At this point I began to appreciate the magnitude of a Mafia vendetta.

I realized that the *LIFE* magazine article had galvanized many against me, the majority being competitors in my own specialty. The perspective on the *LIFE* article, however, varied. For example, a classmate of mine wrote me this letter upon reading the article:

October 31, 1972

Edward B. Diethrich, M.D.
Arizona Heart Institute
St. Joseph Hospital and Medical Center
P.O. Box 2071
Phoenix, AZ 85001

Dear Ted TERRIFIC!

Barbara and I enjoyed reading the recent Life Magazine article.
We're delighted to have a classmate and friend doing so very
well. I hope that everyone understands that your success
is a result of brains, hardwork, and that extra something that
compells a person to take that one step beyond. We're proud of
you and Gloria, keep up the good work.

With best personal regards,

Eugene M. Helveston, M.D.
Associate Professor of Ophthalmology

It seems an ophthalmologist was not threatened by publicity regarding a doctor in another specialty. The jealousy, envy, and viciousness became apparent in the depositions. The hospital had arranged for a group of surgeons from the American Association for Thoracic Surgery to come to Phoenix and review some charts that had been hand selected by my local opponents. Their report was, as expected, not very favorable. However, when Phil and another one of my local attorneys, Ed Hendricks, deposed one of the surgeons on the select committee, Dr. Jay Ankney from Cleveland, Ohio, the case took a surprising turn. Ed called me, "Ted, you thought we might find a smoking gun. Listen to this. Dr. Ankney admits that the visiting committee did not review a single one of the selected cases. Their final opinion was based on personal bias, not upon facts."

That was a blow to the detractors; their "special" agents had been exposed. Yet, I was still facing a hearing with the all-powerful executive committee of the hospital. We were all aware of the pressure that had been applied on them by the angry mob. There was little preparation we could do for the hearings except to pray they would go in my favor, when suddenly I had the idea of contacting Bill Helm, my interviewer for the medical society application. He was friendly to me in our hospital encounters and a member of the hospital executive committee. I called his home and he invited me to stop by that evening for a chat. It turned into a three-hour conversation. It was really the first opportunity I had to speak directly to any of the executive committee members. I spelled out the entire story in detail, and Bill listened carefully, occasionally indicating he had not heard that or this side of the story before. At evening's end, we shook hands and he patted me on the shoulder.

"I am glad we had this conversation, Ted; let me see what I can do."

I will never know if the final decision of the executive committee was influenced by Bill's opinion, similar to the situation with Dr. Coller years ago relative to the interview situation with Dr. DeBakey. Deep down inside I believe it was indeed. Then suddenly, a serendipitous event occurred.

The evening before the hearings, I was studying a few hospital charts on the key patients they might question me about. One of these cases caught my eye because it had attracted international attention a few months before. It was not my intention to tell this story, but when my friend and AHI Foundation attorney Paul Meyer asked if I was going to relate the story of the upside-down valve in my book, I changed my mind.

Many months before the current string of events, Paul and I were battering some balls against the frontenis walls on our lunch break. (Usually we didn't have much time to change clothes before going to the courts, and sometimes we changed in the car, joking about what it would look like in the headlines of the newspapers: "Heart doctor and his attorney caught in car, changing clothes in the sport court parking lot.")

On one of those occasions he asked, "Ted have you ever sewn a heart valve in upside down?"

"Not that I know of. Why would you ask?"

"Well, there is a rumor spreading about town that you did just that and are trying to cover up the mistake. Bill Cornell, a local heart surgeon, made that allegation while delivering a speech at the Rotary Club." I reassured him that I had never made such a grievous error.

We went ahead with the game, but I must confess my mind was blocks away in the operating room. How could such a story be spreading?

I later learned it was spreading like an epidemic. Everywhere I went, even abroad, I was asked about the upside-down valve. As in all these ugly accusations, the truth eventually wins out.

The story is that of a valve implant operation where the patient was not doing well. We were not able to completely remove her from the heart-lung machine. While I was waiting for the heart to recover, I went to the operating room lounge and was speaking out loud about why we were having this problem. Was the heart muscle too weak? Had there been a bolus of air into the heart arteries? Could I have put the valve in upside down? The latter question was not a serious one, but rather a reflection of my frustration with the situation. Later, I learned there was a resident in the lounge during the discussion. I did not even see him in the room. He was the physician eventually discharged for his dishonesty in the research laboratory regarding the Gore graft.

This was a great opportunity for the attackers to further discredit my reputation. The "upside-down valve" was to be the key weapon to assassinate me at the hearing of the hospital executive committee.

As I looked at charts the night before the hearing, I recognized the name of the patient who had a valve replacement problem. It was surely the alleged upside-down case. I carefully dissected the chart in preparation for the next morning.

Their pompous attorney presented the case. They had brought Dr. Barmuda, one of my former fellows, back to Phoenix to testify against me.

"Could I ask a few questions?" I inquired after they made their case. They did not deny me because they were sure the scalpel was already deeply embedded into my heart. I took the medical record and sat it down before their star witness. I pointed to the piece of paper that showed the pressure tracings in the aorta above the valve.

"Does this represent the pressure with the valve sutured in position?"

"Yes," he responded.

"And there is good pressure?" I asked. He looked at me. "Yes."

"Now, this is a follow-up tracing recorded several minutes later. Is there still good pressure?"

"Yes."

"Do you know that this tracing identifies that the heart lung machine has been off for nearly twenty minutes, and there is still a good aortic pressure?" There was a pause before he replied again.

"No, I did not realize that."

"Tell me doctor; could there be any aortic pressure with the heart lung machine off with the valve sutured upside down?" The room went dead silent, and the prosecuting attorney's face turned red. The now-shaking Judas fellow, my former trainee, was perspiring.

"The valve was not sutured upside down," he muttered.

That taught me a lesson. In strange company, be careful with your words. They may be purposely distorted and come back to haunt you. In this case, they could have come back to destroy my reputation. Was it Winston Churchill who said, "Loose lips sink ships?"

My defense team was confident that we would win, and there was the possibility of significant cash rewards for all. The pendulum had swung in my favor. An important letter was sent to the local newspaper from the president of the hospital's medical staff. The local headlines suddenly became positive, and my distracters went into hiding. They would never be my friends, but my very nature is to forgive and forget. That was sometimes easier for me than for my associates.

October 28, 1975

Editor
Scottsdale Daily Progress
7302 E. Earll Drive
Scottsdale, Arizona

Dear Editor:

The Scottsdale Progress published on October 27th, 1975, an article on its first page, by a Preston Long, that has grossly distorted fact and is a deliberate effort to discredit Dr. Edward Diethrich, St. Joseph's Hospital, and its physicians.

The article has taken a few facts and allegations and opinions out of context and represented them as all fact. In addition, the newspaper did not publish any of Dr. Diethrich's replies or defenses against the allegations, etc. I personally believe that the Scottsdale Progress has done a grave injustice to Dr. Diethrich and owes him a public apology.

Whoever gave the newspaper this information has violated Public Law A.R.S. Section 36-445.03 and I fervently hope will be found and be held responsible for this offense. Dr. Diethrich and other medical staff physicians and hospital officials are prevented by this same statute from discussing these matters or any medical audit publicly.

Sincerely yours,

Robert B. Leonard, M.D.
President of the Medical Staff

I had continued to teach daily using new devices and techniques. I had just started a procedure when Nelson Dyess, my chief anesthesiologist, came barging into the operating room.

"Ted, have you lost your mind? Bill Cornell, the very surgeon who lambasted you at the Rotary Club about the upside-down valve, is scrubbing in to see your procedure?"

"I know, Nelson; he called and asked if I could teach him how to do this particular procedure. Please help him put on his gown when he is finished scrubbing."

Nelson said nothing. Just shook his head in disbelief. Another vascular surgeon who had been at the mob country club gatherings called with a similar request that we train his son in our new specialty of endovascular surgery. I also accommodated him. The rides in life are easier if the bumps are smoothed out.

Now that the dust was settling on the suits and countersuits, I had to make an important decision. I met with Paul Meyer, and we had an extremely lengthy

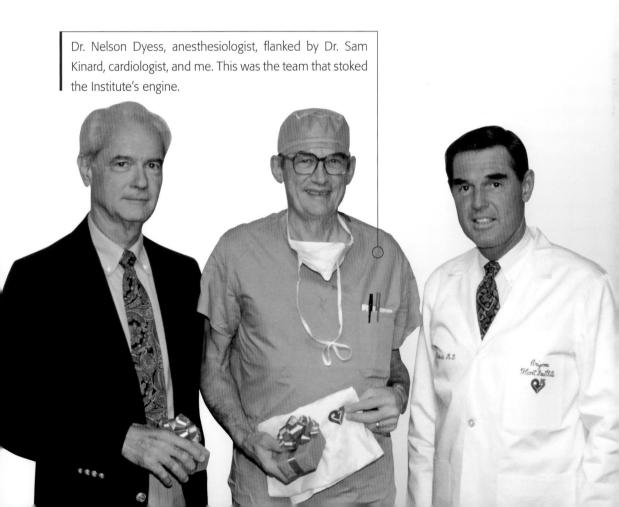

Dr. Nelson Dyess, anesthesiologist, flanked by Dr. Sam Kinard, cardiologist, and me. This was the team that stoked the Institute's engine.

conversation about the future. Paul had been with me since the beginning and, in fact, frequently advised me about strategy.

Would I now continue the war or bury the hatchet and get on with my plans for growing the Arizona Heart Institute? I had been completely exonerated, and it was not a difficult decision. No time to worry about the past; we needed to move on to the future to fulfill our dream. The attorneys were indeed not so pleased with me, but they would have other clients for potentially large cash rewards.

Surgeon Calls Off Suit For $500,000-Plus

"In a statement issued today, Diethrich and the Arizona Heart Institute, which he founded here said:

'The conspiracy case filed in federal court over a year and a half ago by the Arizona Heart Institute and Dr. Edward B. Diethrich against the American Medical Association, the Maricopa Medical Society, several physicians, an attorney and a local hospital has been settled.

The terms of that settlement are not important. What is important is that the parties to the litigation have resolved a bitter conspiracy that never should have occurred and hopefully never will be repeated.

That controversy could not have been resolved in a courtroom without an inordinate expenditure of money and physician time and the resulting public spectacle would not have served the interests of any of the parties, the medical profession or the public. Now that the case has been settled, the physicians involved can concentrate their energies on the more constructive goal of taking care of patients, and the Heart Institute can focus its resources on its continuing educational and research programs which are designed to help *wage a far more important battle—the battle to someday defeat the nation's number one killer, cardiovascular disease.'"*

Whew! I was tired. It would be great to have it over forever. I just wanted to get on with the vision. However, it's clear I still did not understand the Mafia. In spite of my vindication, the one unscrupulous reporter who had led the daily newspaper attack against me continued his assault. In 1990, an astounding fifteen years later, the article "Pioneer or Mechanic" by Peter Alshire really stepped over the boundaries of legitimate reporting. It was clear the reporter's mind had never understood the words "fair and balanced," and neither had the keys on his typewriter.

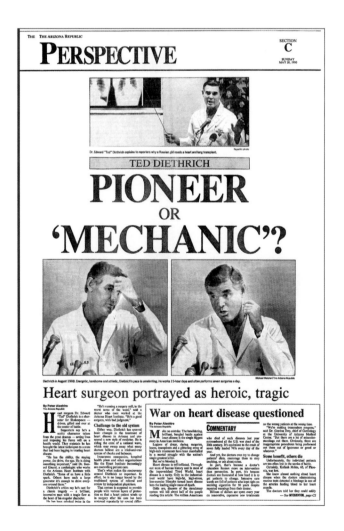

The Arizona Heart Institute staff was outraged. They had a meeting and voted unanimously to respond with a full page, detailed rebuttal to the scandalous article.

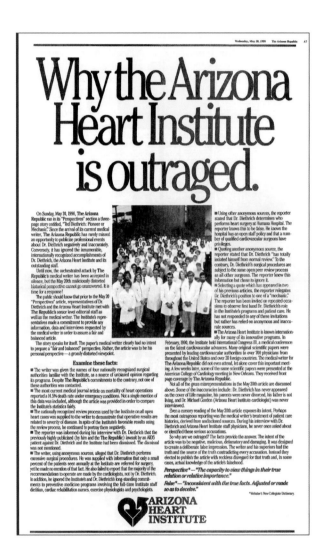

Quite expectedly, the period of the Medical Mafia assault was extremely difficult for me. I should mention that there were numerous calls and letters from physicians across the country who had endured similar attacks on their practices. Frankly, the Medical Mafia problem deserves a standalone publication. It has been written unabridged but not edited and still sits on the shelf at home above my desk.

Another project?

19

"Real Life" at the Arizona Heart Institute

In spite of the tumultuous beginnings and near catastrophes, our program at the AHI was growing rapidly. The space originally allocated at St. Joe's for the Institute was quickly becoming inadequate. We needed more physician offices, patient rooms for clinic visits, and laboratories for diagnostic procedures, especially ultrasound scans and ECGs. All this was high on my priority list, as well as a rehabilitation area for our post-surgical patients. This last space became very important and was soon named the "cardiac conditioning program" to be headed by two of our cardiologists, Dr. Fuad Ibrahim and Dr. Kent Smith. Our program set a new standard of care for post-cardiac surgery rehabilitation. It was so successful that many centers around the country sent their physical therapy personnel to the Institute for specialized training.

In order to accommodate all of these services, we leased a floor at the Del Webb office building a few blocks from the hospital. This allowed our entire program to grow and become more successful. The growth was so great that in 1977, only six years after opening the Institute, we moved the AHI to a new 35,000 square-foot outpatient facility twenty blocks east of St. Joseph's Hospital.

Dr. Kent Smith, founding cardiologist of the Institute's treadmill testing program. Unfortunately, he died young of colon cancer.

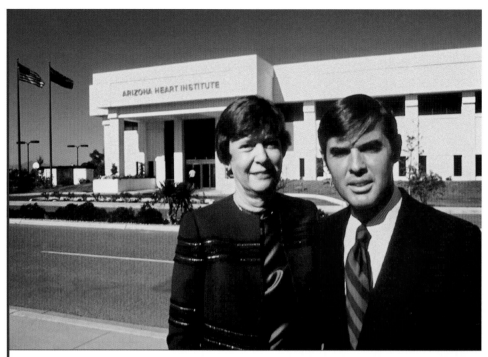

Mrs. Thelma Kieckhefer, board member and major contributor to the Arizona Heart Foundation, standing with me in front of the original Arizona Heart Institute building. This was the site of the first outpatient catheterization laboratory in the United States.

In addition to all the components at the Del Webb office, the new AHI housed a freestanding catheterization laboratory, the first in the United States. This may not seem like a monumental move, but it was just that. Up to this time, when physicians needed to look for disease in the blood vessels by injecting dye and taking a "picture" of its passage through the arteries (angiography), a patient had to go into the hospital. Now, diagnostic angiograms of any part of the circulatory system could be performed in this outpatient facility, which was not connected to a hospital.

I grossly underestimated the medical community's reaction with comments such as "unsafe," "no operative backup," and "a patient could die in transit to the hospital if an emergency occurred." The outcry: "This time Diethrich has gone beyond the cutting edge." Again, this was not only a local response; it reached from coast to coast and beyond. (Currently, this outpatient format is the gold standard throughout the world. In fact, in our own community, vascular surgeon Dr. Phil Wall has three clinics, each with complete imaging capability for interventional procedures.)

In spite of the controversy regarding the outpatient catheterization laboratory, the AHI moved forward in creating an overall delivery system to accomplish its mission of early cardiovascular disease detection, thus enabling intervention to correct, alter, or halt its progression to disability or even death. It seemed like a gigantic endeavor; however, when broken down into components, a systematic program was developed. We called it cardiovascular screening, CVS for short.

We had the ideal setting for this concept: an outpatient facility completely equipped for advanced diagnostic testing and a staff schooled in the knowledge of how to perform a variety of tests with the assurance of the highest quality. I strongly supported the CVS program, which ultimately made a significant imprint on the delivery of cardiovascular care.

I made it a point to introduce this new delivery system whenever I could interject it into a talk or conversation about health care. I remember answering a call in the middle of the night. The voice on the other end of the line said, "This is the White House in Washington, DC, calling for Dr. Diethrich. The medical doctor wishes to talk to him."

The call was not entirely surprising because a few weeks before I had visited the White House while attending a medical conference. The physician wishing to talk to me had spent considerable time asking about the concept of the Arizona Heart Institute, its capabilities and clinical results. He must have been impressed because he proceeded to explain that the reason for the call was his desire to refer his patient to me for a coronary bypass operation. The patient was John Scali, a well-known ABC News

John Scali, U.S. Ambassador to the UN flanked by AHI staff.

THE WHITE HOUSE
WASHINGTON

December 9, 1996

Warm greetings to the staff, volunteers, and friends of
the Arizona Heart Institute as you celebrate your twenty-fifth
anniversary this year.

For a quarter of a century, the Arizona Heart Institute has
helped to lead the fight against heart and blood vessel disease.
You can take pride in your long list of achievements, including
the first heart/lung transplantation in Arizona. I commend you
for providing the highest quality care and for offering comprehensive diagnostic testing. Your hard work and commitment have
enabled you to stay in the forefront of advances in cardiology.

All of those who are responsible for the success of the
Arizona Heart Institute have earned the respect and trust of a
grateful community. Your long-standing dedication has helped to
save countless lives and give comfort to many.

Congratulations on reaching this milestone anniversary, and
best wishes for continued success.

Bill Clinton

White House letter. One of the many contributions that John Scali made to the Foundation
was his endorsement of our programs as witnessed in this letter from the White House
signed by Bill Clinton.

correspondent and then U.S. Ambassador to the United Nations. We discussed the details of the case and within a week the Ambassador's coronary artery bypass was performed. The screen on Times Square flashed the news of the Ambassador's operation in Phoenix, Arizona. He had made a quick recovery, and John and I became good friends. He joined our Institute's International Advisory Board and later introduced me to television and radio host, Larry King, which led to my appearances on his show.

The Ambassador was a perfect example of the ravages of atherosclerotic disease. Not only did he have the

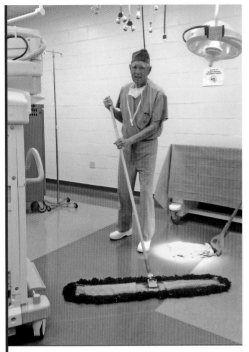

When the OR team was lagging behind, sometimes I had to take matters into my own hands. Even today, as I travel to operating rooms around the world, I don't hesitate.

coronary artery bypass operation, but later a plaque in his carotid artery had to be removed and an abdominal aortic aneurysm repaired. I never knew whether it was too much stress of being a news correspondent or the frustration with the assignment of the United Nations that was the contributing factor to his medical conditions. Probably both. John was no doubt at least partially responsible for the congratulatory note from President Bill Clinton on the 25th anniversary of the Arizona Heart Institute.

When I was in town I operated every day, always beginning around 6 a.m., sometimes even earlier. I would complete the major portion of the procedure and one of my associates would come in to wrap it up and close the incision. This freed me up to go to the Institute for my morning clinic, soon to be known as the EBD Clinic. This clinic was unique in several aspects. I, even though a cardiovascular surgeon, would see every patient in consultation, sometimes more than forty in a

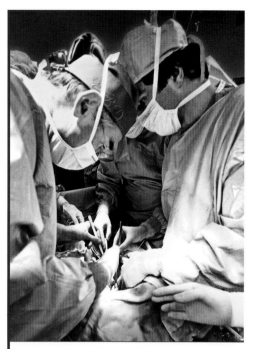

Dr. Ilhan Bahadir, my senior surgical associate and good friend.

morning. It did not matter what the patient stated as a chief complaint, my role was to screen and then triage to the appropriate section of the Institute. Many patients were referred to one of our cardiologists in attendance, which ultimately contributed to the success of this system. In my screening, I ordered the appropriate tests to expedite a thorough workup for each patient. This system was so finely tuned that a new patient could complete several diagnostic procedures, even a cardiac catheterization, all in a single day. At other facilities, this could take a week or longer, with many appointments being scheduled. The fact that everything was under one roof at the same location added greatly to the clinic's efficiency.

The CVS program generated patient information that could be identified and characterized into patterns. These individual components became known as risk factors. There were other investigators in our field who were studying the applicability of these trends in the prediction of heart disease. We conceived the idea of compiling these risk factors in a form, which allowed the Institute's physician to explain to a patient his/her risk of developing heart disease, all based on the results of their diagnostic tests.

This risk factor analysis was condensed into a short list of questions. The answers could be scored, and the total was related to the participant's risk of heart disease: low, medium, or high. This questionnaire then became the basis of the nationally televised "Great American Heart Test."

This segment of the 1981 ABC News "20/20" program was unprecedented for two reasons. It marked the first time that television had been used to conduct a heart health survey, and it drew the largest audience response of any show in ABC News history.

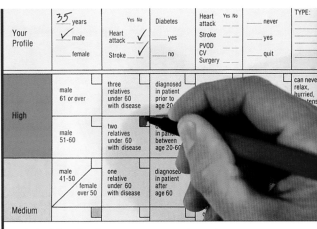

Original "20/20" Heart Test questionnaire.

More than 250,000 pieces of mail were delivered to the Institute. They sent in their scores and questions on the back of old envelopes, scraps of paper, pieces of cardboard, paper plates, whatever they happened to have handy by the TV. One family, while eating a box of Valentine candy, took the test on the lid, realized their own risks, threw out the rest of the candy, and sent us their score on the empty box! These viewers were not promised any prizes, coupons, or a preventive program for reducing their heart risks. This was a demonstration that the American public was thirsty for information, eager to learn about their health, and also what could be done about it. Although caught somewhat off guard by the deluge of responses, our team sprang into action, mounting a tremendous volunteer effort to read, analyze, and respond to each survey.

As moderator, the famous news anchor Hugh Downs indicated we will never know just how many viewers actually took the self-assessment test and discovered their risk for developing heart disease. Probably never before in the history of medicine had so many Americans been aware of their own personal risk factors that could lead to heart attacks and strokes. Long after the "20/20" program, many people continued to inquire about the facts of heart disease and requested more information from the AHI.

A representative from the publishing company Simon & Schuster contacted me after the ABC News "20/20" telecast and suggested that a book be written on this subject. The end result was *The Arizona Heart Institute Heart Test*, published in 1981, just ten years after the Institute's inauguration!

Fast forward to 2014. I turn on the television while shaving, and an advertisement appears across the screen promoting "Life Line Screening Services," and

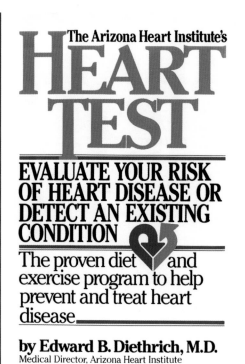

Arizona Heart Test book cover.

the list includes "Stroke Screening, Heart Disease Screening, Congestive Heart Failure, Carotid, Atrial Fibrillation, Abdominal Aortic Aneurysm, Peripheral Arterial Disease and High Blood Pressure." My only comment: Why has it taken so long to bring this science to the surface? Could it be related to the dollar bill and will economics influence the future?

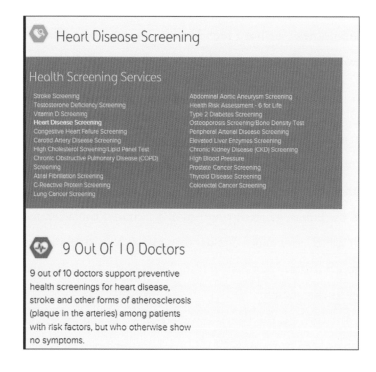

20

Up Close and Personal

I t was 1998. I was having my carotid arteries scanned with the duplex ultrasound technology we had been advocating in the CVS program at the Institute when a calcified plaque (lesion) was found in my right carotid artery. It was not a significant narrowing, and I had no symptoms. The protocol under these circumstances was to repeat the scan at six-month intervals, which I did regularly.

One morning about three years following my initial scan, I left the operating room and returned to my office in preparation for the EBD Clinic. I took off my surgical cap and was combing my hair when I suddenly noted a loss of vision in my right eye. It was not just blurred; I could only see through my left eye. I brushed my hair again and walked carefully down the steps to the clinic. By the time I reached the ground floor I knew I was in trouble. I made my way to the nursing control desk, and motioned to the head nurse to follow me into an examination room. I closed the door.

"I have amaurosis fugax* in the right eye," I confided. "I'm blind in that eye, and I think I'm going to have a stroke. Call the operating room, locate Dr. Rodriguez (my senior associate), and tell him he will need to perform an emergency carotid endarterectomy as soon as possible."

Can you imagine the concern of the staff? By the time I reached the holding area next to the operating room, my vision in the right eye had nearly returned to normal. The staff prepped me for the operation. Dr. Rodriguez appeared at

*A temporary blindness that may result from an insufficient blood supply to the carotid artery.

the doorway, and his expression was a combination of disbelief and confusion. No one had told him that the emergency operation he was about to perform was on Dr. Diethrich.

Think of this scenario: if I had never had a carotid scan and therefore not known about the calcified plaque and its potential consequences, I would not have called Dr. Rodriguez. At that point, there would have been no diagnosis. Was it a tumor? Had a blood vessel ruptured or maybe a blood clot moved from the heart to the carotid arteries? Multiple tests would have been ordered, all costly and with significant time delay. The end result could have been much less than favorable. This single personal episode convinced me of the value of screening in spite of its inherent cost. It's an argument that is still current among my colleagues, as well as insurers and patients who pay for these tests.

21

Breaking Ties with St. Joe's Hospital

As successful as we were at St. Joe's, with the outpatient cardiovascular screening and conditioning laboratory in the rented space at the Del Webb building, and later at the AHI building, it became patently obvious that our program had several shortcomings. One of these was the need for additional funds to support research and education. A logical source was the hospital. Abner Huff was the administrator, so I approached him with a request for $200,000 a year to support these activities. He turned me down without any conversation or thought of discussing my request. I calculated that there was something very wrong with this equation. We were bringing in millions of dollars per year to this hospital, and they could not find a way to support that small request for research and education?

That evening I sat in my study at home. I had the 8½ x 11-inch lined pad on the desk. Although I was not sure what direction my thoughts would lead me that night, the pad and pen were always with me whenever I was in an intensive, pensive mood. Suddenly, it dawned on me. In spite of the distractions with our success there had to be some hospital in the Valley that would welcome our services. I turned the pad horizontally and began on the left, listing hospitals in the Phoenix metropolitan area from west to east. At that time, the furthest west was Boswell Memorial Hospital. About in the middle on the pad was St. Joe's. I drew a strong black X over that name; they were never going to be a true partner. I then moved a few blocks to the east, and there was Doctor's Hospital. It was an unusual facility,

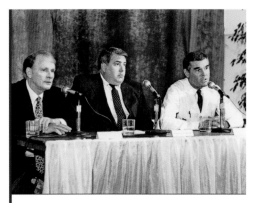

David Jones of Humana Hospital System, Raymond Rouleau, (Humana administrator), and me, announcing the AHI program at the Humana Hospital in Phoenix.

privately owned by a small group of local physicians, mostly general practice (GP) physicians and general surgeons. The major shareholder was Dr. Allen Ginn Jr., of the GP group. I knew him well because he was one of my referring physicians for heart operations at St. Joe's. Early the next morning I made the phone call to Allen. I was straightforward and simple: "Do you believe there would be any interest in having the Arizona Heart Institute at Doctor's Hospital?" I asked. He responded that he had no idea, but he could find out soon.

It was mid-morning when one of my employees, Paula Banahan, RN, Executive Director, ran into my office.

"You have to come to my office immediately. I have David Jones, head of Humana in Louisville, Kentucky, on the phone," she said. "He has reviewed our Request for Proposal and has only one question: 'Where do I sign?'"

Racing back to her office, my mind began to formulate the possibility that the Institute may actually find a new home, and that's exactly what happened. The lawyers from the hospital and Paul Meyer from the Institute took care of the details. We were leaving St. Joe's, and in one year from the date of signing our new agreement, we would be operating in a new facility.

Without going into great detail, Humana opened its arms to our team and its checkbook to our programs. They directed millions per year to the Institute for operations and marketing expenditures. They renovated the small Doctor's Hospital with more than $25 million in new bricks and mortar and capital equipment to complete the facility and welcome the new AHI team. Each existing department received a facelift, and where there was no department, one was created. The total cost was a far cry from the measly $200,000 we had requested from St. Joe's.

Canine Friends

Dogs have always been a part of my life. You may wonder at the dichotomy: How could I have dogs for pets and yet use dogs in research? What helped me through it was the knowledge that the research animals were contributing to the development of new treatments for cardiovascular disease. I never lost my affection for those early "patients." My experiments with rabbits were only a brief interlude in my canine affair. Today, most animal research does not use canines; pigs, sheep, and other animals have become the choice for experiments. If computer simulations improve, the need for animal testing may soon be a thing of the past.

Would it surprise you to know that throughout the last forty years I have had four golden retrievers, their names all reflecting one of my life's triads: Harmony, Symphony, Cadence, and Tympani.

After we had moved away from St. Joe's Hospital, it was apparent that many patients in our new hospital were missing their own pets that were at home. We initiated a "dog therapy" program; a canine greeter and I would make rounds, and the dog would lie on a towel placed on the recovering patient's bed and show affection.

Cadence—a Wolverine rooter!

As a component of our dog therapy program, I brought my golden retriever Cadence to the office each day with me. She would greet staff and patients while I was in the operating room. Each Thursday we had a 7 a.m. staff meeting in the large classroom, and Cadence would cross the hall from my office and see what type of breakfast rolls were being served. None was on her diet.

When the presentation began she would sit quietly next to me, looking at every slide as if it were in "canine lingo."

On occasion, when the lecture was boring or running way over the allotted time, she would sit straight up and give a loud, disapproving bark, very uncharacteristic of her behavior. She must have felt an impulse from her master's aggravation with the presenter.

Unfortunately, she developed an auto-immune disease when she was seven years old and in spite of all the medication and treatments, it was hopeless. I knew it was near her end. The morning after she was put to sleep, I put her picture on the screen at the end of the staff conference.

"Cadence went to canine heaven last evening, but she wanted to thank everyone for their friendship and putting up with her occasional stealing of a donut off the chair of one of the attendees," I told the staff. On that sad morning, I needed a little dog therapy myself. Many staff members sent me condolence messages, and some even presented flowers. Just another reflection of how the AHI Team operated as a strong unit.

The thought of losing Cadence and not having a companion in my office on a daily basis was not acceptable. I instructed my secretary

Cadence in the office preparing for the CV conference across the hall. She never missed a session or the breakfast rolls that were served.

to initiate a US-wide search for golden retrievers, with emphasis on availability of a female puppy. She did a great job and found a breeder at Centennial Ranch in Platteville, Colorado, just north of Denver.

The woman's name was Anne, and she and her daughter each had litters due on January 6, 2008. It was perfect timing; I was scheduled for a meeting in Denver around that time, and with only a slight readjustment, I made plans to visit the puppies. It should only take an hour or so.

Arrangements made, I rented a car in Denver and drove to Anne's farmhouse. It was not exactly what I expected. It seemed like there were dogs everywhere, and maybe of every kind. Nevertheless, she greeted me and was very sweet and proud of her golden retriever puppies running around the living room and kitchen. There were maybe a dozen or so, and even with all the dogs in my life, it was the first time I had actually gone to pick one from a litter. It was impossible; they were all so cute!

After an hour or so she asked if I wanted to drive over to see the daughter's litter. What could I say? In essence there was no choice—let's go! I don't know what I was expecting, but it was a perfect duplication of the first scenario. Now I have twenty or so puppies from which to choose in two different farm houses.

After another hour of confusion and my inept skills in puppy canine selection, I asked if I could see the first litter again. Of course—and back to the mother's house we drove.

Now, I knew I couldn't keep this up all day. My allotted time was running short. So I repeated the assessment of each puppy, and in near-exhaustion I lay back on the living room floor. That's when I saw the puppy come up the kitchen steps, heading straight for me. She crawled onto my outstretched arm and settled on the floor with me. Canine drama over! I did not pick my dog, my dog picked me.

I was disappointed to learn that I could not have the puppy for six to eight weeks, but it was just as well. In seven weeks I would be going to a yearly conference conducted by Jim Margolis, MD in Snowmass, Colorado, where our condominium is located. I could pick up the puppy on my way and have seven or eight days for puppy training. Who cares about a medical conference when a new puppy has arrived?

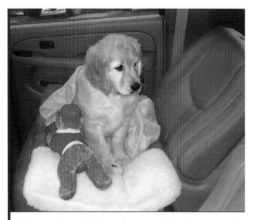

Tympani settled in the car after the transfer in Vail, Colorado.

We made arrangements to meet halfway between Platteville and the Denver airport. Anne would bring the puppy to an appointed coffee house, and I would pick up the dog and head on to Aspen. She even brought an extra blanket and a toy for the puppy. The transaction only lasted a few minutes before I was on my way to ski with my new canine companion. Halfway to Aspen, at the freeway exit near Vail, I stopped for a cup of coffee and a potty break for the puppy. I had already begun her training. As I came out of the Dunkin' Donuts with my coffee in hand, my cell phone rang. It was my secretary.

"Catastrophe! Catastrophe!" she said, panicking. I was certain something horrible had occurred at the hospital. "You have the wrong dog! You have your puppy's brother!"

What was I to do? I wanted a female golden retriever, yet I was already in love with the male pup. No, I could not have two dogs, so we arranged to turn around and meet the mother with my puppy at a nearby roadside restaurant.

We met, made the transfer of brother for the sister, and I was calm and kind to Anne. Even in human circumstances, such things happen. Have you ever heard of the nursery switch? Well, hopefully not too often. Back in the car, I now had the female puppy on the seat next to me. It was the beginning of a new life together.

A couple of years later at the University of Michigan Cardiovascular Center Advisory Board meeting in Ann Arbor, I told this "ice breaker" story. One of the members looked at me and said so simply, "Ted, did you ever think of turning the puppy over?" Isn't that a lesson for life? Turn things over and take a second look!

Tympani sporting her new AHI attire for the pet therapy program.

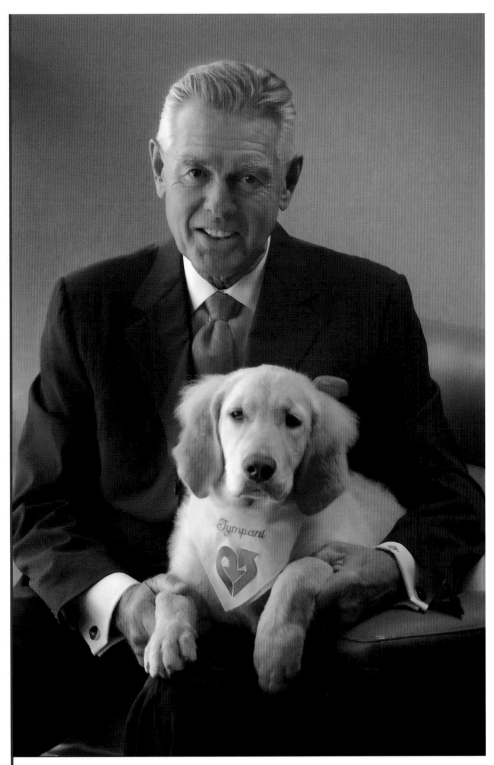

Tympani in her pensive mood.

23

Is it a Boy or a Girl?

One of the research areas I was pursuing in the 1970s was the development of ultrasound technology, with an initial focus in cardiac echocardiography to assess heart function and valve status. While at the American College of Cardiology meeting in Dallas, I was strolling down the commercial exhibit area with Dr. Joe Futral, a cardiologist who had gone through our training program and was practicing in northern Arizona, when he nodded at a fellow approaching us along the exhibit lane and said I should meet him. That's when he introduced me to Marty Wilcox, an engineer that lived outside of Denver. He had a lab set up for his developmental work in his garage.

We sat down for a coffee and soon agreed that we had similar interests. Over the next several months we met frequently and discovered various opportunities in the echocardiography arena. There wasn't a great deal of money required for this initial phase of our work. It was mostly assembling various pieces of equipment and testing the imaging results. Individuals who needed some electrical connections assembled for another project had contacted Marty, and that job provided us with some money in the pot. I knew as soon as the echo project took hold, he could abandon that part-time work. We met for an update session whenever I was passing through Denver, and on one of these occasions, he pulled a Polaroid photo from his jacket and bluntly stated, "This is my new unborn baby boy!"

My response was passive, demonstrating my lack of knowledge in the exact science of this field. "How do you know it's a boy?"

"Marty, can you really tell the sex of your unborn child?" I asked excitedly, my voice rising.

"There it is in the picture," he replied, pointing again.

Although I was attempting to control it, I am sure my enthusiasm was obvious. Finally I said, "Marty, you are a millionaire!"

It was obvious that the little Polaroid photo represented a gigantic

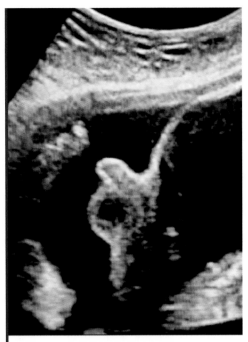

Male embryo—ultrasound study identifying the sex of the unborn baby.

opportunity for the future development of a company. We selected a name: Advanced Diagnostic Research (ADR for short). That name seemed broad enough to represent whatever idea or pathways we might want to pursue for the future. We leased space in Tempe, Arizona, and established a small company that initially had almost exclusive emphasis on obstetrical ultrasound technology.

We were the original company to provide an examination to validate the sex of a fetus prior to birth. It eventually became very lucrative, and we were in fact the first ultrasound company in this business. Obviously, I do not need to emphasize the interest this company created worldwide. After several years we sold ADR and moved on to other areas in the cardiovascular field.

I never lost my interest in the ultrasound technology. In fact, I started an ultrasound school at the Arizona Heart Institute and Foundation in 1982. At that time the major emphasis was on cardiac ultrasound, but I was moving rapidly in the peripheral vascular area with our new technology and the ability to obtain high quality contrast studies in the new hybrid OR arena. The combination of noninvasive examinations documented with the contrast material was an important step in our endovascular program. When we opened the school, Terry Reynolds, BS, RCDS, was hired as its director. His initial emphasis was cardiac echo sonography, but over time I convinced him peripheral had to be a strong component of our program. That has turned out to be entirely true since most job positions today in this field either are now, or will be in the near future, requiring training certification in both modalities.

I am extremely proud of the school's development over the years. The accomplishments of the school and its current success in both educating students and placing them in positions attest to the long tradition of program excellence of the Arizona Heart Foundation. This science is on the cusp of the next major quantum leap in the 21st century. Don't blink. You might miss it because it is present just around the next curve. In fact, in Eric Topol's new book, *The Creative Destruction of Medicine,* he provides an exciting prediction of where imaging will make a dramatic restructuring of how we diagnose and care for patients. Here is how he describes it:

The date was December 27, 2009. That evening, I had just gotten my hands on the first pocket-sized digital imaging device that provides high resolution imaging in the United States—the Vscan.

Until this point, the only way to get an ultrasound of the heart, an echocardiogram, was to send patients to a lab, where they'd be studied with a $300,000 machine the size of a refrigerator. This was an exciting and liberating event. Naturally my first step was to image my own heart.

To get the images is quite simple. A transducer, which has the shape and size of an electric toothbrush with no brush, is placed on the chest after some gel is put on its tip to help transmit the ultrasonic energy. The transducer is moved around the chest to find a good "window" to acquire digital movie loops of the heart in multiple standard views, each revealing something different about the heart muscle function, the thickness of the heart's walls, the status of the four heart valves, the size of the four chambers, how the segment of the aorta near the heart looks, and whether there is any fluid in the pericardium (the sac around the heart).

Placing the transducer on my chest, I quickly got a crystal clear image of the main pumping chamber—the left ventricle—and the mitral valve. I was not surprised that my heart muscle function looked fine. But then I put the color flow on, which uses ultrasound to track the blood flow, and it showed that my mitral valve was leaking badly—so badly in fact, that I had just become a potential candidate for open-heart surgery to repair the valve! I finished the rest of the ultrasound exam of my heart, and everything else was OK, with the minor exception of a moderate leak from my aortic valve. (At least that one wasn't severe enough to warrant surgery). The whole scan had taken less than five minutes, and even most of that was taken up by the shock of seeing, and repeatedly examining, my leaky mitral valve.

It just didn't make sense. I had been feeling well and exercising vigorously almost every day. I knew, however, it's possible to have a slow, insidious, progressive leak without showing any symptoms. So I got out my stethoscope to see what I could hear. I listened to my heart in various positions, and I could hear some leak from the valve, but it sure didn't seem like much—maybe 1+, on the cardiologists' scale of 1 to 4, but not the 3+ the Vscan showed. It was peculiar, but the Vscan was tracing the blood flow, and I was looking right at it—lots of leaks and enough to be requiring a consultation with a heart surgeon.

Pocketsize, high-resolution ultrasound is one of the most significant advances in medical imaging in decades and is replacing the stethoscope, which has been around since 1816. I now use it to examine every patient I see in clinic, and it usually preempts the need for another appointment for a formal echocardiogram study. It not only saves time but a lot of money (a combined technical and professional charge of about

The GE handheld Vscan.

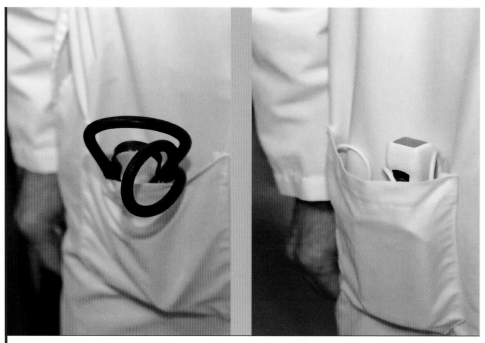

Comparison of a stethoscope and the Vscan in the pocket of my white lab coat.

$1,500 per echo). With over twenty million echocardiograms done per year in the United States, there's certainly room to improve efficiency.

Dr. Topol's personal experience and his justified enthusiasm for the ultrasound discipline coincide with the projections for the Arizona Heart Foundation's ultrasound school. One of the objectives of the school currently is to bridge the gap that exists between the high tech devices and the practical application by the healthcare providers. Education will be required, safety precautions initiated, protocols developed, and certifications put in place. Presently, these issues may only be at a superficial level. I see our ultrasound school taking a major position in rectifying this void.

Serendipity just keeps appearing everywhere.

24

Video Arts Studio

My experiences in both Michigan and Houston emphasized and reinforced my commitment to an audiovisual department in the new Arizona Heart Institute. I considered it vital, not only for both public education and scientific documentation, but also the dissemination of our work worldwide. We established a department named Video Arts Studio (VAS) and employed both medical illustrators and cinematographers. (Keep in mind that this was still in the era of 16 mm movie film.)

A special boom was designed and constructed so that the cinematographer could be directly over the operating table. It was a close copy of Dr. DeBakey's boom in Houston, plus a few more bells and whistles. However, the cameraman in Houston was in a sitting position while our cameraman was lying on his abdomen.

The single event that catapulted VAS' reputation overnight was the first live case presentation of an open-heart operation on television in 1983.

Dick Williams, head of VAS at the time, had been working with Arizona State University School of Television. A variety of plans were suggested to increase public awareness of heart and blood vessel disease. One that was of particular interest was the idea of showing a live open-heart procedure on television. The telecast would be accompanied by a discussion of risk factors for coronary artery disease, alternative treatments for heart disease, and suggestions on how to reduce

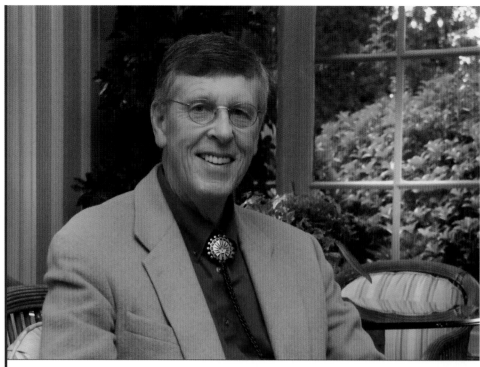

Steve Harrison, aka "Leonardo" was Director of Medical Communications at the Institute.

the risks. Dick approached me with the idea. We had done numerous surgical films together, winning many awards for these presentations.

The idea of "live" was not a big variant in what we had done before; in my teaching of students, fellows, and residents, the procedures were often live with an active question-and-answer discussion. I had never considered this to impair the operator's performance or add an increased risk to the patient.

Dick proposed to Ted Christenson (assistant station manager at KAET, the local PBS affiliate) that we enter into a venture between the Arizona State Board of Education, AHI, and KAET. The idea was to involve the various school districts throughout the state in the study of the cardiovascular system, culminating in a special evening event of a live heart operation from the Arizona Heart Institute via the KAET broadcast network.

After a few days, the assistant station manager came back with a counter suggestion: we should cut out the school idea and just do a live operation during

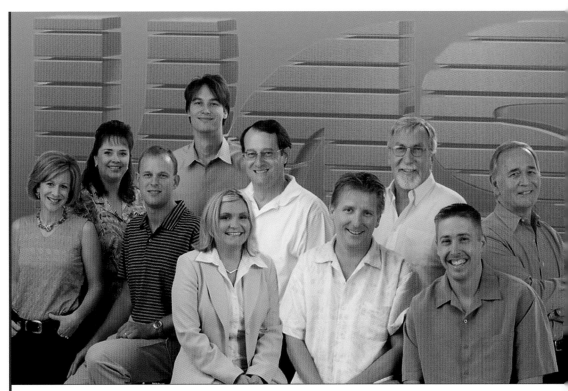

VAS staff in the 1990s, from left to right: Marisa Maggio, Harelson PR; Yvonne Smith, graphic designer; Mike Austin, medical illustrator; Nathan Greene, web master; Kristen Conant, PR; Jim Burk, business manager; Chris Wooely, managing producer; Keith Kasnot, art director; Wayne Dickmann, video producer; Richard Williams, marketing director.

Heart Month to KAET's statewide audience. Although somewhat disappointed in not doing the more altruistic educational idea, I accepted the challenge, and the planning for the event began. A procedure was scheduled for February of 1983.

During my planning, while flying back from business in Chicago, I contemplated the amount of effort being applied to the event and the limited audience it would reach. I had an idea and called Dick for a meeting. Why not go national or even beyond? Heart disease was not confined to Tempe, Arizona.

Station manager Chuck Allen suggested that Ted Turner might be willing to donate satellite time, which would make the broadcast available to the nationwide PBS system. I responded enthusiastically to KAET's generous offer and detailed planning continued. The possibility of satellite time and nationwide distribution continued to be a factor in the planning, even though it wasn't confirmed. Funding was needed, and we were still waiting to hear about Ted Turner's donation.

One week prior to broadcast, Dick informed me that Turner was not going to come through with the satellite time donation. I asked Dick how much money we were talking about. "Three to four thousand dollars," he replied. I knew I couldn't let the money stand in the way of national coverage. I called a few "well-positioned" friends and within minutes the additional cost was covered. I instructed Dick to proceed with the plan. It was to be a telecast on PBS nationwide and our local Channel 8.

The unique feature of the telecast was the perspective provided via the overhead boom to the viewer, which was identical to the surgeon's view. When discussing the procedure with a few lay people before the telecast, there was a feeling that it was going to be "gory and bloody." In fact, except for the blood in the tubing of the heart-lung machine, the audience barely saw a drop of blood.

News coverage included *USA Today*, *Los Angeles Times*, and ABC's *George Strait*. *TV Guide* even labeled "The Operation" as one of its "best programming" shows of 1983. In Great Britain (BBC), viewers enjoyed the operation during their afternoon tea and scones.

One of George Strait's questions to me in a press interview after the operation was, "Why did you do the operation live rather than tape it?" My response was, "For the same reason your TV producer put 'LIVE' in the upper right-hand corner of the TV screen during the broadcast." It was real time; no delay or edited action as the surgeon and his team were creating it. He was quick to challenge.

"But what if something goes wrong?"

"Like you, we can always go off the air," I said half-heartedly. In all my years, however, I have never had to resort to that exit strategy.

I never anticipated that George's questions were only the beginning of a barrage from every angle.

"Unethical," "irresponsible," and "non-professional" were the terms used in letters, comments, and medical journal editorials. What I thought had been a great

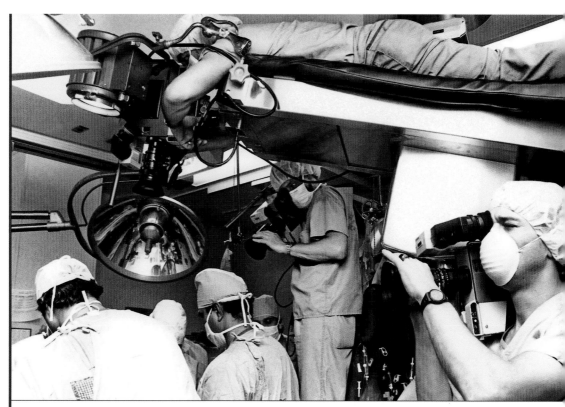

The overhead boom designed at AHI to provide a live, birds-eye view of the heart operation. Notice the cameraman lying flat for more precise filming.

service to the public, informing them about heart disease and hopefully alleviating the fear of procedures like coronary artery bypass, turned out to be a crusade against "live" operations, which persists today at many levels. Major medical meetings have sessions dedicated to discussion and debate on this issue. Even the FDA has taken the position that no device under investigation for clinical approval can be shown in a live telecast without special permission. This will continue for some time since live telecasts are standard practice throughout the world today. It's just that we did it first, taking the brunt of the attack in paving the way for the future.

Like the varying opinions of the *LIFE* magazine article, from condemnation to admiration, the live open heart procedure was either vilified or exalted; it was all in the eyes of the beholder. For example, recently I was invited to give the keynote address at the Southern Vascular Society meeting in Phoenix, Arizona. Dr. Ali

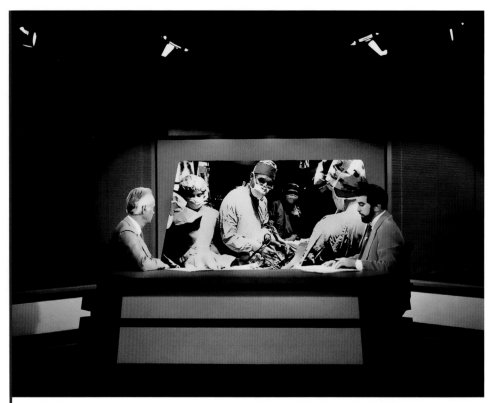

Speaking to Richard Dalli, host of the live open heart operation on Channel 8, with Dr. Sam Kinard moderating.

AbuRahma, President of the Society, was the moderator. When introducing me, he referred to the live televised operation.

After completion of my general surgery residency and while applying for a vascular fellowship, I remember it like it was yesterday. I went to my late Chairman, Dr. James Boland, and asked his thoughts regarding the vascular fellowship offers I had received. Without hesitancy, Dr. Boland advised me to immediately sign on with Ted Diethrich of the Arizona Heart Institute. I remember him telling me that when he was in Dallas during his thoracic fellowship at Southwestern University, he went to Houston to observe Dr. Michael DeBakey's technical skills, and to his surprise, he ended up observing Dr. Diethrich instead of Dr. DeBakey. Dr. Boland was very impressed with Dr. Diethrich and felt he was the most talented and technically skilled surgeon he had ever seen and, therefore, Dr. Boland strongly encouraged me to go to Phoenix for my vascular fellowship. I think my decision was also influenced when I learned that Dr. Diethrich had been invited to Jordan to perform the first open heart surgery on a VIP Jordanian, and he was then awarded the Medal of Independence from King Hussein of Jordan. This award is apparently given to the scientist who makes the greatest contribution to the people of Jordan.

In addition, although he doesn't receive much credit for it, is the statement used by some of my past visiting professors, specifically the late Jim DeWeese, who visited us in Charleston, West Virginia, over two decades ago. When Dr. DeWeese discovered that I had trained under Dr. Diethrich, he reminded me that one thing he admired about Ted Diethrich, which was the reason he invited him to be a visiting professor at the University of Rochester in New York when he was the Chief of Vascular Surgery, is that Ted had done something that no one had ever done before—perform a coronary artery bypass graft on live television, which was broadcasted on public television networks all over North America. Dr. DeWeese felt that for someone to do that on live television 2–3 decades ago was unthinkable at a time when people felt that this procedure was so difficult and complicated, but Ted made it seem so easy for the public to understand.

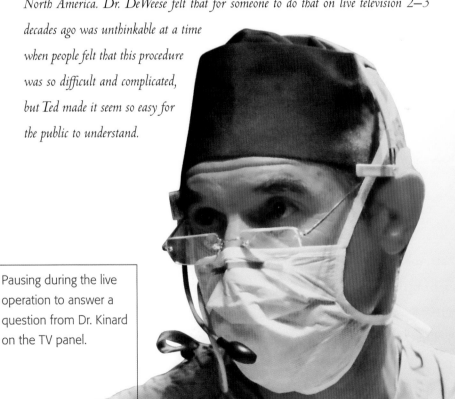

Pausing during the live operation to answer a question from Dr. Kinard on the TV panel.

25

Silence is Golden

One morning while scrubbing, a visiting student asked me a peculiar question: "Why don't you have music playing while you are operating, Doctor?" Indeed, I had visited numerous surgeons who spent considerable time selecting the music they wanted played in the operating room during the procedure, maybe more time than planning the operation. The more I thought about that inquiry, the more it appeared that I had a paradox in my life and work.

Music has been an important element in the triad, and here I had eliminated it during the periods in which I spent most of my waking hours. On the other hand, I did have a good explanation. The performance of an operation demands complete attention to the details, not to be disturbed by music blasting out of wall-mounted speakers, which by the way were nonexistent in my operating rooms. So, I provided the student with some interesting surgical history.

In the early days, why were operating rooms called operating theatres? It was because they were amphitheaters, and the onlookers peered down to the center where the operation was being performed. Usually, the chief surgeon had an assistant (or even several) surrounding the patient, so the view for the students and trainees was not exactly spectacular, certainly not like from our overhead boom!

This separation of the operating physicians and the onlookers also provided a yet unknown "sterile" environment. It was not until after Joseph Lord Lister (1827–1912) introduced bacteria to the world that operators were required to don caps and masks. Simultaneously, there was a rule of silence evoked in order to reduce the spread of bacteria through communication; hence, the protocol for silence in the operating theatre.

To further reduce verbal communication, the surgeon and surgical nurse passing the instruments communicated only by hand signals. The surgeon would give a particular signal, like spreading the first two fingers, and the nurses would place a scissor in the palm of his hand, sometimes with a rather theatrical motion. In those days, learning

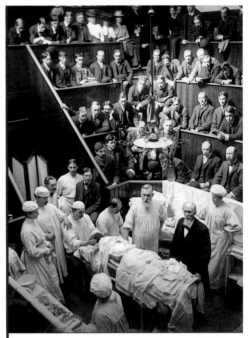

Classical amphitheatre for demonstration of operative techniques.

surgical sign language was part of standard training, but today it is a lost art. This was probably more information than that student expected, but the value of silent communication would soon be appreciated in another operative setting. We were preparing for a heart transplantation. A local TV station had requested to film the procedure for educational purposes. I spoke to the director before going to the operating room. There were some aspects of this filming request that were troublesome to me. Something was just not right; what was their motivation? I smelled a problem but could not put my finger on it. It was enough concern that I delayed the operation a few minutes so that I could speak to the entire operating team, nurses, technicians, and doctors very privately.

It was impossible for me to provide much explanation for my uneasiness, because I did not have my own concerns synthesized. I had the option of canceling the case, throwing out the TV crew, or evoking the rule (absolute silence) throughout the procedure. I know that sounds like an impossible command to execute, but I have just explained the hand signal routine.

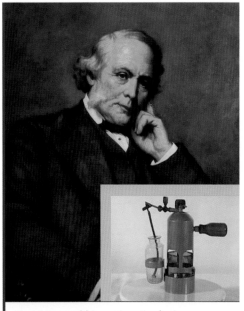

Dr. Lister and his antiseptic device.

You must remember this team operated together every day, often from 5 a.m. until dusk. There was an unparalleled skill set and a standard of discipline that had been created from within. They did not question my decision.

In reality, the silence mostly affected the operating team at the table, which is where the TV crew placed the microphone, and conversations could be broadcast. The entire transplantation was performed without a word spoken between the surgeon and the nurses. No music in the operating theatre; the smooth motion of the team and the maneuvers of the surgeons created the melody. A dozen Bose speakers could not repeat the performance of those maestros. After the procedure, my conviction that they were up to no good was further confirmed.

What they didn't tell me was that they heard a rumor about the status of the donor's heart, which had provoked their interest in this procedure. They were told he had a long history of drug abuse, and a reporter said that Dr. Copeland, a transplant surgeon in Tucson, Arizona, had turned down the patient as a donor. Later, it came out that drug abuse was not the reason, but rather it was unsuitable for any of his current patient recipients. When we used the heart, the story the press created was along the lines of "Surgeon transplants poor hearts." The patient lived two years, and at the time of his death the story was reprinted, neglecting to say the cause of death was cancer.

26

It's All About Teamwork

During my days in Michigan and later on in Houston, I had little time for my interest in sailing. However, Joe Morris, my mentor from Michigan, had a small sail boat, and he would invite me to join him during the weekends. Later on, he and I bought a Thistle number 101 and towed it from Perrysburg, Ohio, to Ann Arbor, Michigan. It was a great hobby, and I had it in my mind that one day I would become a serious sailor.

Ironically enough, this dream turned into a reality after I moved to the desert. In Phoenix, the summers were hot, and the ocean wasn't too far away. My son, Tad, was equally interested, so we purchased a sail boat equipped for racing; it seemed like everything had to be a competition.

While VAS was primarily a medical audiovisual department of the Arizona Heart Institute, I didn't limit it exclusively to medical work. As it turned out, sailboat racing was a natural fit for VAS films. If you have witnessed America's Cup, you can appreciate its thrilling action.

We were doing a campaign with my boat *Triumph* including the Victoria Maui Race, which we won, and the Transpac, in which we were far from being the winner. The MEXORC Series, which was far more drinking tequila than competitive sailing, led us into the Panama Canal crossing and on into Antigua. We had the VAS film crew on most of these excursions, although not during the Antigua Race, where we were headed onto Sardinia and then the English Channel.

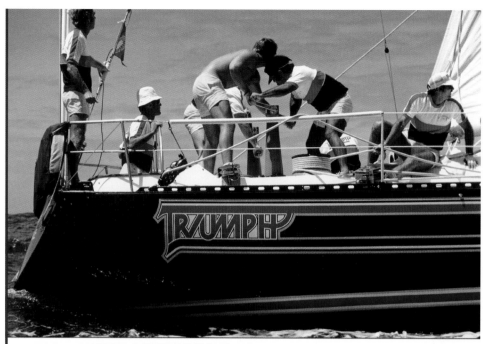

Our boat, *Triumph*, equipped for emergencies.

Racing in the English Channel off the Isle of Wight was a new experience for most of the crew on *Triumph*. A few had raced in San Francisco on one of our competitions, where we tackled a race course around Alcatraz and faced the changing tides under the San Francisco Bridge. The currents in the English Channel however, were so complex that I had made arrangements for a navigator, one very experienced in the area's racing conditions, to join our crew. The major challenge is the point during the race when the tide changes and we had to make a 180-degree directional adjustment. The racecourse committee had this programmed perfectly. Interestingly, the opening of America's Cup World Regatta in 2015 was hosted on the same waters around the Isle of Wight.

As we approached the buoy the navigator instructed me to go around and at that point the crew deployed the anchor. *Triumph* was facing the outgoing tide; we were not going anywhere…just sitting there quietly. Well, not really so. As we looked at all the yachts in a similar position, one stood out. It was Prince Phillip's yacht, part of the racing regatta. *Triumph* crewmembers quickly went

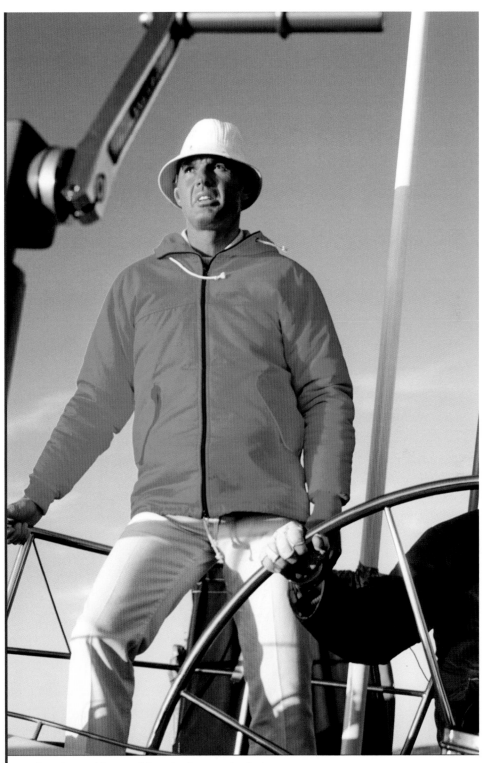

My favorite position: Guiding the boat at the helm.

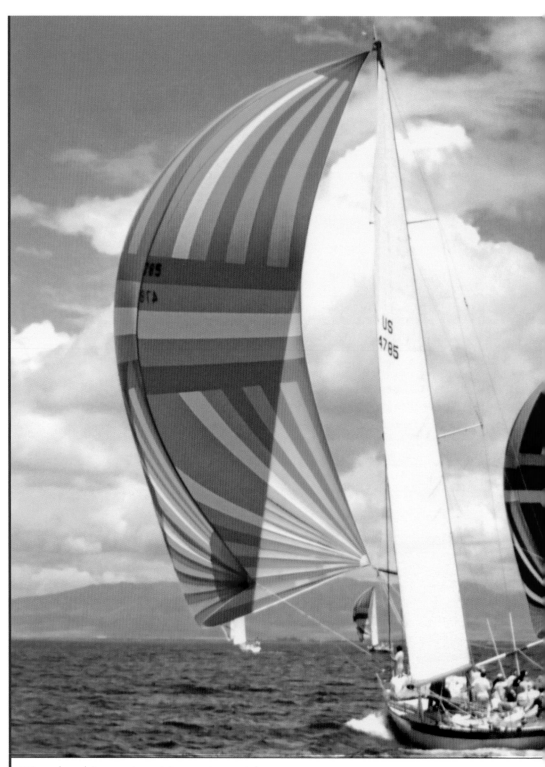

Triumph and *Sorcery* in a vicious racing match.

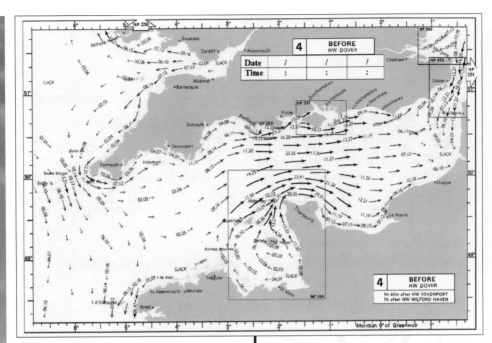

Map showing currents of the English Channel, a tricky place to race.

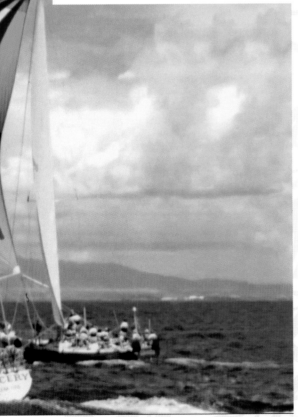

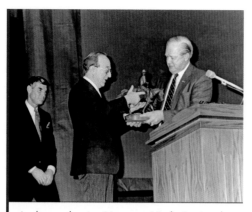

Ambassador to Norway, Mark Austead receiving a bronze sculpture in recognition of his many contributions to the Arizona Heart Foundation Board. He also narrated the award winning film, *Man Against the Wind*.

below deck and surfaced with a dozen or more white Frisbees with the *Triumph* logo. My crew had apparently spent some late nights in the pubs with the Prince's crew because they seemed to know them and started calling back and forth to each other. Then the *Triumph* Frisbees began to soar toward the Prince's deck. One by one they fell short; not one reached its designated target. We were all disappointed by our ineptitude at that game. No Frisbees came our way from the Prince's yacht.

A month or so after the race, back in Phoenix, I sent a letter to Prince Phillip with a *Triumph* Frisbee enclosed. I explained that our crews had enjoyed each other, and we wanted to present this small gift.

Surprisingly, I received a letter from the Prince, thanking me for the Frisbee and acknowledging the crews' camaraderie. He wished me good luck in future races. I did not make Frisbee skill tests as part of my *Triumph* crew's selection process.

Our biggest event was the Pan Am Clipper Cup Series in Hawaii. This was a large Regatta, but the special thing to us was the match racing. *Triumph* was a CC 61-foot sloop. A similar boat named *Sorcery* from California made this a natural racing challenge for the skippers and crew. The racing conditions, with strong winds, were perfect for big boats.

The crew arrived five days before the race in order to practice under these conditions. I had the VAS film crew prepare a documentary of the entire event under Dick Williams' direction. Dick placed a camera on our challenging boat *Sorcery* to capture dialogue between the crews. In preparation for this book during 2014, I reviewed the final film product from the Clipper Cup Series, which eventually aired on public television. A former US ambassador to Finland, Mark Austead, narrated it.

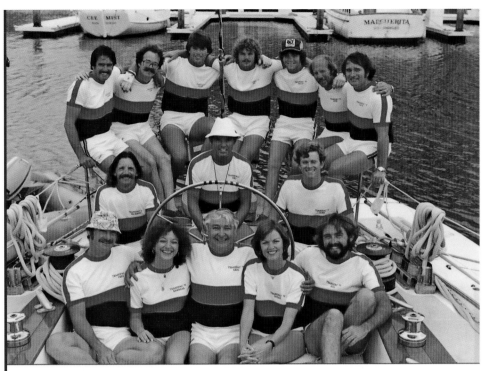

Creating the *Triumph* team.

One of the things that became very clear in my research for this book is the remarkable pattern that repeats itself in my life story. Building a structured, successful team is something that I've always strived to accomplish.

In the operating room where there was strict discipline, image, and dress were just as critical. Perfection was demanded regardless of what it might take to achieve. (Sounds reminiscent of my early experiences with Dr. Szilagyi and Dr. Revelli and later on with Dr. DeBakey.)

The same was true for sailboat racing. I had special uniforms made in Hong Kong, with different shirts for different races. I have always used the analogy that when the Green Bay Packers race onto the football field, their uniforms are all the same, from helmets to socks. Even their shirts are tucked in. I felt the same way about our racing team and *Triumph*.

When crossing that starting line, I wanted the team to look like they were all members of a well-honed racing team, and I wanted the boat to look like a sleek

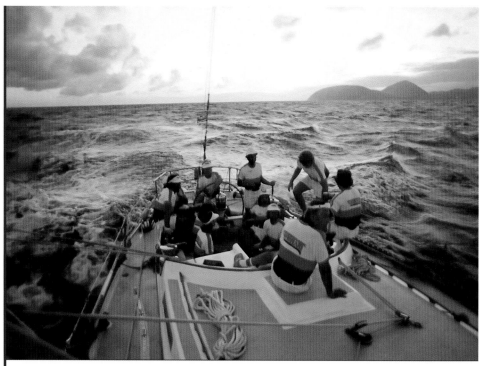

One of the joys of sailboat racing.

racing craft. The way we painted it, the way we kept the boat up and the entire team in uniform, is just part and parcel of reflecting the teamwork that goes into making a winner!

Each crew member had a particular position. For example, my son, Tad, manned the bow of *Triumph*. Because of the heavy winds, we needed sixteen crew members, some mostly for ballast. We practiced sail changes until they were perfect. I was not going to accept a mistake in deploying the spinnaker. The cameraman recorded a firm lecture I gave to the crew: "You guys are doing exactly what I told you not to do, you know! You better start slowing down, giving quiet orders and telling guys ahead of time what to do or it's going to be chaos."

It's all the same in my mind, no matter the activity or task you're engaged in. This is why our operating team performed like a team, which was obvious when the cameras rolled to capture hundreds of the surgical procedures we've performed over the last forty-five years. It's all like a symphony, with the conductor providing direction to his team. As in the operating room, sometimes all the practice in the world cannot prevent an untoward experience.

An event that exemplifies this is the video narrator describing the stretch race in Maui: "Now *Sorcery* and *Triumph* are neck and neck, heading to the finish line. The only thing now is to hope their luck holds out. Just when *Triumph* is giving everything she's got, when every sail is trimmed to the max, a shackle holding the jib lets go and for *Triumph* the finish line might as well be a thousand miles away."

However, when we crossed the finish line in the final race ten boat lengths in front of *Sorcery*, I knew all the hard work was worth it. The effort that goes into building a successful, functioning team is a repeated theme in my life that cannot be denied. My own personal reward was to organize the transformation of a disparate group of fellows into a winning team.

27

Old Glory, Upside Down

With my medical background, I was predisposed to safety on board *Triumph* and incorporated a stock of medical supplies and equipment for any emergency. We established an aggressive racing campaign, one where crew members arrived a day or so before the race for practice. After race day, the crew returned to their jobs until the next race. I had one secretary who did all the scheduling, and one of my OR nurses was in charge of the medical supplies. As proof of our protocols, safety and man overboard procedures were rehearsed. I could have done an appendectomy on board if there was a need for one.

The most major surgery performed was suturing a very large scalp wound on our Captain Ricardo's head. Fortunately, there were never any broken bones, but everyone knew the doctor's yacht *Triumph* was a good ship if an emergency should ever occur, and it did!

We were racing in Antigua for the big boat series. A boat named *Glory* was our toughest competitor. After two days, we were nip and tuck, heading into the last leg of the closing race. *Glory* rounded the buoy three boat lengths ahead of *Triumph*, but I wasn't too worried. The wind conditions favored *Triumph* on this crucial leg. I was at the helm as usual, looking ahead at *Glory's* stern. We were definitely gaining. In fact, it seemed that *Glory* was slowing down and sailing off course. Suddenly, I saw two of her crew at the stern holding the American Flag upside down: the signal of an emergency on board.

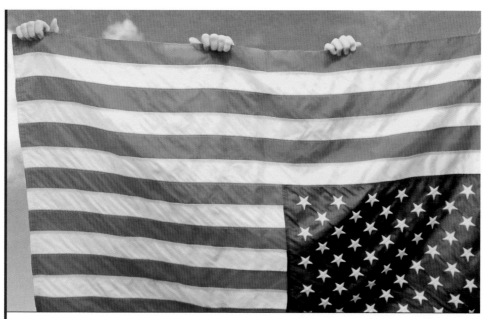

Old Glory flying upside down is never a good sign.

"Drop the sails!" I yelled to the crew. "Yes, all of them!"

I turned on the engine and steered at full speed directly toward the emergency. At the same time I instructed Captain Ricardo to go below and bring up all the emergency supplies. He and I would have to board *Glory*, and I wanted everything ready since there was no telling what the catastrophe might be. We pulled alongside and boarded, and there at the foot of the mast lay one of the sailors.

I quickly learned he had suddenly collapsed while pulling on the line. A quick examination told me this was bad news; he was not breathing, and had no pulses or blood pressure. We started an IV, and used an ambu bag for respirations in addition to chest compressions. In spite of all the support and medications, it was apparent that this young sailor had suffered a catastrophic event and quickly died.

I instructed my crew to go on with the race. I would stay on *Glory* and head back to the harbor to meet the officials and explain the situation. I was not familiar with the regulations or procedures, since I had never had a crew member die on board. The next morning the police visited me, and I was relieved that they were assured there was no foul play regarding the event.

About three weeks later when I was back at the Institute, I learned more about the death. This fellow was known to have Marfan syndrome* and took medication for hypertension. He was under treatment at a medical clinic in Los Angeles for an ascending aortic aneurysm. The autopsy showed the aneurysm had ruptured, and we could not have saved him even under the best of medical conditions, certainly not mid-ship at the mast of *Glory*.

I learned several lessons that day. No matter how much we practice and what preparations are made, adverse situations will be encountered that are beyond our control. Even *Triumph's* resuscitation equipment and a cardiovascular surgeon at the helm were no match for this man's pathologic condition. While winning the race has always been paramount to me, it is put in a different perspective when a human life is lost.

Never again do I want to see Old Glory upside down.

---

* *Marfan syndrome: A hereditary condition causing blood vessel expansion, which eventually can lead to aneurysm rupture.*

28

Monte Carlo

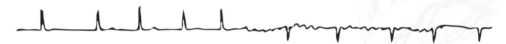

I made a practice of going to my office in between operations while the next patient was being prepped. It was just off the corridor of the operating room, and it gave me an opportunity to call the referring physician to give a progress report on his patient. I could also check the schedule with my secretary and return phone messages, which were always plentiful.

On this particular day, she said that a Mr. Wilbur Stromberg from the Loews Corporation in New York City had called about a medical matter. I did not recognize the name and at that time was not familiar with the Loews Corporation. I instructed her to put the call through, and a friendly Wilbur immediately answered. He stated his matter was not a business call, but rather a personal call in regards to his brother's heart condition.

He described it as desperately severe coronary artery disease and added that no surgeons in New York (the city where his brother lived) were willing to accept him for operative therapy due to his extremely high risk. It did sound like a high-risk situation to me, but I said I would see him in consultation without any commitment to surgery. (This is the short part of the story.) We operated, and he most fortunately had a very good result, considering his condition could have meant dying on the operating table. On the contrary, he recovered and went back to work.

Wilbur was overwhelmed with appreciation. He began to call me so frequently that my secretary would just say, "He is calling again." However, one time in

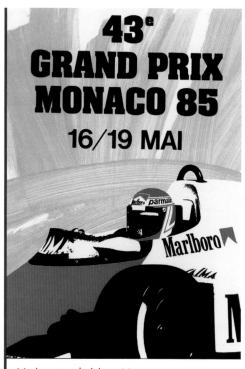

43ᵉ
GRAND PRIX
MONACO 85
16/19 MAI

Marlboro

My inaugural visit to Monaco.

particular he was not calling just to say hello and chat. He wanted to see when I could join him as his guest in Monte Carlo, where he and Henri Lorenzi were in charge of building the new Loews Monte Carlo Hotel in the small municipality of Monaco, a historic spot for the Grand Prix Formula I racing.

After many invitations and an equal number of rejections, I could not pass up the Pan Am (Super Sonic Charter) invitation from New York City to Nice, France, during the month of May. He even extended the invitation to include any physician colleague I wanted. I contacted Dr. Dino Tatooles. (He was the one who had helped me with that loading dock incident in Chicago when I was a resident.) I explained the opportunity to him, hoping maybe we could develop a future program together in that location.

The plane was filled with executives going to the hotel's grand opening. Of course at that time I did not know any of them, but Wilbur was a most gracious host and made me feel very welcome. That same ambiance continued upon arrival at the hotel, although the activity level was several decibels higher. I met Henri Lorenzi, the head of the hotel, and he was quick to introduce me to a number of his very important guests. What I had not anticipated was the role he wanted me to play. I am sure it was not planned; it just happened as with most serendipitous events.

There were some important guests and employees as patients who were admitted to the local hospital for a variety of medical conditions, and Henri had no compunction about asking me to go "visit/consult" on some of them. I was actually eager to help. It was in fact an opportunity to see what medicine was like in this small section of the world. Needless to say I did not operate, but rather confirmed the treatment and reassured the patients. It was a rewarding experience; one that I thought would be once in a lifetime, but that was not so.

For the next several years, Wilbur insisted that I attend the race along with my pal Dino. I never envisioned the experiences that ensued, or the impact they would have on my medical career.

On one of those trips a few years later, Henri found me at lunch on the roof restaurant. He asked if I could see one of the hotel guests, and of course I jumped up and followed him

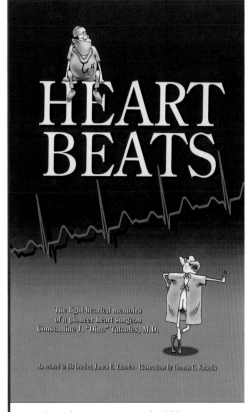

My friend Dr. Dino Tatooles' life story.

along the rows of chairs next to the pool. He stopped and introduced me to the "patient," and it was none other than the famous trumpet player Al Hirt, who was also known as Jumbo, for short.

I examined him and found a non-life threatening condition. He had a tender, reddened area in the lower right calf; it was superficial thrombophlebitis. We chatted for some time, and once he learned that I played the trumpet in the Michigan Marching Band, he seemed much more interested in me. After a couple of days with leg elevation, heat, and rest, he was

Dino and me embracing at the signing of his book, *Heart Beats*.

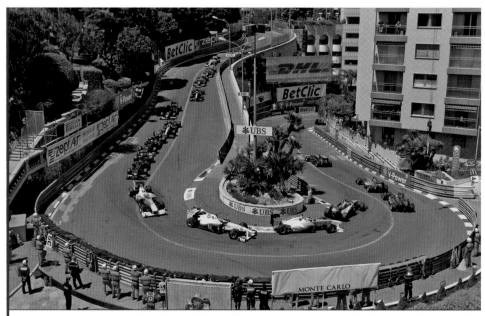

The famous hairpin turn at the Monte Carlo race.

back to normal. We stood together watching the race machines turn the famous circle in front of the hotel.

I never expected to hear from Al again, so it was a real surprise when I opened a box a few months later and found a thank-you note: "With much appreciation. Enjoy playing this special trumpet, Al." Indeed, I did, and whenever I was in New Orleans, I visited Al at his club.

Among the many people I met in Monaco, one of the most interesting was Leopoldo Pirelli, the president of Pirelli Corporation and the grandson of the company's founder, Giovanni Battista Pirelli. We became very good friends over the years, and when he required vascular surgery to correct blockages in circulation to his lower extremities, he came to see us at the Arizona Heart Institute. We also had a parallel interest in sailing, and during the big boat series in Sardegna, he hosted my crew in his mountainside villa. The *Triumph* sailors considered that a real treat after the so-so meals coming from its galley.

Medicine, sports, and music, that inseparable triad, consistent with my proclamation to Uncle Ken: I was made for work, not play.

29

AHI Abroad

The introduction to important and interesting people did not end with Al Hirt. Wilbur had many friends and contacts that were quite rich and influential in the region. For example, he invited me to dinner with Mario Contini, one of the hotel's investors, who I had the opportunity to tell my story of the Arizona Heart Institute and my plans for the future. He asked about the possibility of a similar heart institute in Monte Carlo. I was interested, but at the time my plate was pretty full. Eventually, there was the establishment of a cardiovascular center sponsored by the Prince and Princess of Monte Carlo. I visited that center and observed the work they were doing, which was quite impressive.

Several months later I received a letter from Mario asking about the possibility of me visiting a hospital in Modena, Italy, where he had ownership. He wanted my opinion about further investment in the facility. By coincidence, the following week I had planned to visit Europe for a medical meeting. It would be a minor deviation to visit the Hesperia Hospital in Modena. In truth, I looked upon this as just a courtesy visit, where my input on the project would have little impact.

Upon arrival the chief executive and medical officer of Hesperia, a private general hospital, greeted me. I was escorted to the third floor conference room, where snacks and champagne were served. After a glass of champagne and some social chatter, they took me on a tour of the hospital. As we passed through the first floor, I noticed a large area under construction. Upon questioning I learned they

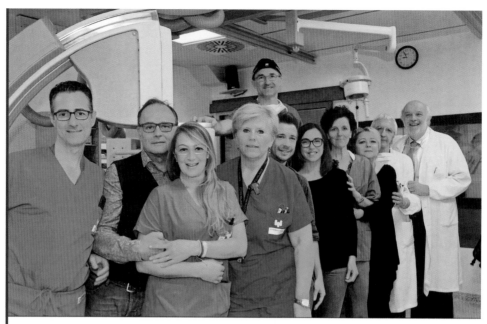

Dr. Alberto Benassi, far right, and his team at Hesperia Hospital in Modena, Italy—site of many of my endovascular interventions and techniques.

were building two new operating rooms and an intensive care unit. I immediately shifted my mind-set from a brief local visit to a potential professional opportunity in research and education. I expanded my tour and spent nearly three hours there before departing for Venice, my next scheduled stop. On the drive my mind was turning over the possibilities for the hospital I had just visited.

Right after checking in I placed a call to Mario Contini in Monaco, expressing my gratitude for the opportunity to visit his hospital in Modena. The formalities were brief because I wanted to present my proposal. In my mind it was simple and entirely logical, but could I convince the owner?

"Mario, you are building new operating facilities. If you would permit me to design the operative area suites to mirror ours in Arizona, including the imaging equipment, I would be prepared to visit the hospital each quarter to teach and do research with new techniques and equipment in the rapidly growing field of endovascular surgery." His response was immediate. "Let's meet and initiate the plans for the program. It sounds great to me."

Then I called Steve Hanson, my partner in Interventional Surgical Systems, an imaging business we started in 1988. It was going to be an incredible opportunity to move research ideas forward without the constraints at home in the United States.

Many physicians had come from Europe to train with us in this new field of endovascular surgery, later

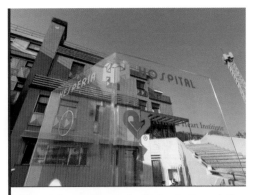

The Arizona Heart Institute & Foundation logo is displayed on a sign at the front entrance of the Hesperia Hospital.

called endovascular therapy. I relied on these friends in establishing the Modena program. Alberto Benassi was the Chief of Cardiology at Hesperia Hospital in Modena and an expert with interventional skills. He had developed a well-knit team that was very receptive to assisting me in performing these new procedures.

Further south in Salerno, Italy, Giancarlo Accarino was developing a peripheral vascular practice, which offered the potential for many patients to be referred to Hesperia. Not far from Modena was the town of Ferrar, where Dr. Stefano Manfrini, who had spent several rotations with us in Phoenix, was eager to participate in the new technology. A third member of our team was Konstantinos Papazoglou, nicknamed "Papa," from Athens.

We had a very efficient system set up. When a date was selected for an operative trip to Hesperia, I would notify Alberto and Giancarlo. They would make the arrangements for the patients and the operating schedules. The OR team had several carts with equipment labeled "Dr. Diethrich's." Much of this represented projects in progress because we were prepared to treat arterial problems from the neck to the foot. It was not uncommon to operate on ten to fifteen patients over a day and a half to two days.

Earlier in this book, I mentioned the need to change the anesthesia arrangement when we opened AHI at St. Joseph's. Well, it seems anesthesiologists can be difficult on both sides of the ocean. At Hesperia I encountered a problem with the "gas passers"

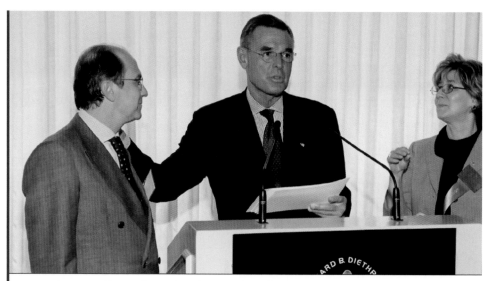

Presenting a certificate of membership into the Edward B Diethrich Vascular Surgical Society to my good friend and colleague from Salerno, Italy, Dr. Giancarlo Accarino. At my right is Erika Scott, Society Administrator.

(an uncouth name for anesthesiologists). We needed to use two rooms whenever possible in order to complete all of the procedures, which meant increasing the tempo of the team. I found that giving the anesthesiologists a little extra oxygen was helpful.

In 2013 we celebrated the 16th anniversary of the Modena Hesperia Hospital program. Some of the technology now used commercially in the U.S. and around the world was first developed and tested in this program. For example, two endografts used for exclusion of aneurysms, both in the chest and abdomen, were first tested at that location. We were very active in using stents in the carotid arteries and focused on better methods of their delivery with specially constructed catheters. Many of the patients had significant arterial problems in the lower extremities.

Dr. Papa and I had developed an endograft to treat these specific arterial blockages. The technique was eventually transferred to the Arizona Heart Institute where the results were confirmed in a scientific publication. There are many more examples, but the key element of the Hesperia story is how much science and product development can occur when a team of specialists has an opportunity to embrace unencumbered creativity and excellent support facilities.

30

White Angels on Cycles

While many of my medical encounters in Monte Carlo were initiated by consultations, there were others that came about in a surprising (or serendipitous) manner.

My interest in sailboat racing had alerted me to a special sail and equipment store in Nice, which was only an hour or so ride away on motorcycles. Dino was not so interested in the sailing part, but the ride along the coast sounded very exciting. We awoke early the day of the planned trip, only to be met with cloudy skies and some mild raindrops. However, we made an executive decision to jump on the bikes and head to Nice.

Soon after departure the sprinkles picked up, and by the time we reached Eze, we had rain but no rain jackets, just our white cotton bike jackets, which were traditional but not rainproof. We were forced to pull into a gas station in hopes the rain would subside. This produced a considerable delay in arriving at the boat store. Our new projected arrival time would coincide with the typical French lunch period, and as a result the shop would be closed.

By the time we arrived in Nice we were not hungry, but it seemed that a beer was in order. Afterwards we climbed on the bikes and headed toward the main shopping area of the city, relieved that the weather was improving. Once we felt that an appropriate amount of time for the French lunch period had passed, we went back to the parking stand, jumped on the bikes, and headed toward our sail mission.

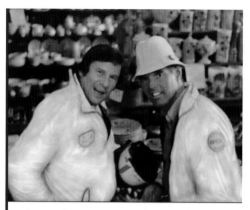

Dino and me in the apothecary shop.

Suddenly, at a stoplight, I heard a child screaming and saw a woman pulling him across the intersection. I yelled to Dino as I looked at the apothecary sign on the store where the child was being dragged. It looked like a serious situation. We laid the bikes on the curb and raced into the pharmacy.

The child was lying motionless, face up on the floor, the mother crying her eyes out. Almost nobody else was present. Without communication we quickly lifted the child to a low counter. Dino began mouth-to-mouth resuscitation and I initiated cardiac compression. He was not breathing and was without pulses. The pharmacist looked on without a word, and employees gathered around as we worked feverishly over the boy.

As more and more bystanders approached, I looked at one and said in English, "Call the ambulance, this child is dying."

Dino was totally engrossed in the respiratory resuscitation, and I put my right index finger on the boy's right carotid artery. Suddenly, I felt a definite pulsation where before it was absent.

"Dino, Dino, keep it up. He is coming back!"

"He's breathing and moving," responded Dino. I looked around the apothecary shop, now filled with people who surely weren't there for prescription refills. Some looked at me with a very quizzical gaze, while others smiled, looking relieved. The ambulance, and what would be called the paramedics today, arrived. The boy was fully responsive, with a good pulse and normal breathing. Then, I assessed the situation.

There we were in a foreign country, no medical license, maybe a hint of beer breath, surrounded by... who knows?

"Dino, it's time to leave. He's in good hands; head for the bikes."

We walked out the front door, passed through the crowd, crossed the corner, and started the engines for our trip to the sail shop. Mission accomplished, and a

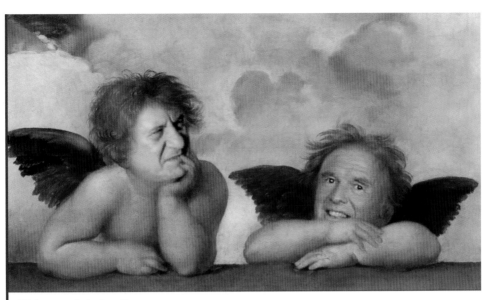

White angels indeed!

positive result. What if there had been no French lunch period? We would not have stopped for a beer and intervened in the apothecary life survival.

We looked at sails briefly before heading back to Monaco. Somehow the thought of sailing did not seem quite so relevant after the apothecary episode.

The next morning as we were sitting with our cups of coffee, Henri Lorenzi, the hotel manager, stopped by our table. He had the morning addition of the Nice newspaper in his hand.

"There is an interesting article in today's paper titled, 'Two Motorcyclists Save Small Boy's Life,'" he began. "According to bystanders, two motorcycles driven by men in white jackets were stopped at the intersection waiting for a light change when a mother carrying her child across the street was yelling 'My child is dying, my child is dying.' She entered the apothecary shop, and the cyclists witnessing this put their bikes on the curb and rushed in behind the lady.

According to the pharmacist, "the child appeared lifeless. No motion or breathing. The men in the white jackets went immediately into action. They placed the child on the counter and initiated cardiopulmonary resuscitation. They obviously knew what they were doing and had been trained somewhere. They did not speak French but spoke to each other in English. I called for an ambulance. After a short period, which seemed like hours, I could see the lifeless body show some color. I heard the one fellow say to his partner, 'Keep it up, keep it up. I feel a pulse.' Then a minute or so later in an excited voice, 'We got him back, we got him back.' The boy began to breathe and started to move his arms. By this time my shop was crowded with onlookers. The ambulance arrived, and I began explaining the whole episode to the attendants."

"When I later turned around to thank the white-jacketed fellows, they were nowhere to be seen. A lady at the front door confirmed that the gentlemen had left the shop, climbed on their bikes and motored down the street. Who were these white angels on cycles that saved the little child's life?"

Henri looked down at me wryly. "You guys wouldn't know anything about this, would you?" We kept our heads down and continued eating our oatmeal. What if we had elected to cancel the ride to Nice due to the poor weather? What if the rain had not slowed us down, and we made it to the sail store on time? What if we had not paused for a beer near the Apothecary shop? What if we had not taken and lived by the Hippocratic Oath?

You can call it whatever you want: Being at the right place at the right time, fate, coincidence, or destiny? But serendipitous or not, I believe it is a residual of the Christmas Day sled wreck.

31

An Artist and Surgeon Join Views of Open Heart Surgery

My 1974 book, *Code Arrest: A Heart Stops* was never a best seller; the same goes for my 1994 book, *Women and Heart Disease*. I like to think that society was just not quite ready for either of those topics. Today, there is a book a day on health and heart disease, and it has become fashionable even with Hollywood. However, *Code Arrest* did turn out to open a serendipitous opportunity.

After reading the book, an executive from the Young Presidents Organization (YPO) called me. The YPO is comprised of young company presidents who, before the age of forty, have created million dollar companies.

The executive asked if I would be available to speak at one of their national conventions. Of course I was excited to do it—not necessarily to promote the book, but rather to make a connection with such a prestigious group of business people. Their mode of operation beyond the national meeting was a series of regional meetings throughout the world. I joined the tour circuit, and right next to me at almost every event was the famous artist LeRoy Neiman. I had purchased many of his paintings of sports and animals, which are still in my house collection to this day. Since LeRoy and I would connect every several months at these events, we became friends, and gradually I initiated conversations about him doing a painting for me. Because of our mutual interest in sports, I thought frontenis was the natural. Never been done before, uniquely different, international flavor, how could he resist?

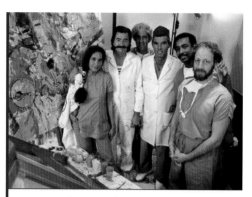

LeRoy Neiman and our surgical gang in the dome during a quiet break in his work.

"Ted, I'm a little burned out on sports and animals right now," he admitted. I could understand that, because they were abundant in my personal collection. I moved on to another non-painting conversation. It was not the right time to convince him on his future art work.

Several months passed, and the scene repeated at a dinner prior to one of our presentations. "LeRoy, I have been thinking. You need to do something in an entirely different arena…not the bullring, not the African safari. Go for a differentiator, the operating room."

I thought LeRoy was going to choke on his steak.

"No way Ted. You are not going to get me into a heart operating room." That initiated a conversation that lasted at least an hour. "LeRoy, you can't imagine the beauty of the human heart. The color is unbelievable. Repairing a problem with the heart is like restoring a master's painting. No one has ever done 'The Heart Operation' on canvas. If you are worried about being nervous or nauseated, I'll have meds for you." Needless to say, it took more than one dinner to convince him, but over a period of time, he began to grasp the potential magnitude of this opportunity.

On the Sunday he arrived in Phoenix, we were having a social gathering of the Foundation board members at my home. LeRoy stopped to say hello before he and I went to the hospital. I took him into the empty operating room and explained the equipment. Then, upstairs to the dome that looked into the operating room below. It was there that he would set up his equipment.

We had a schedule: He would arrive in the dome at 8:30 a.m. each day, and I would come up to chat with him in between operations. He would have lunch, resume work, and leave at about 4:00 in the afternoon. I would go up to the dome before he left to see if he had any questions; usually there were none.

Then late one Thursday morning the circulating nurse said LeRoy wished to talk to me. I went up to the dome while the surgical fellow finished closing the chest.

LeRoy announced that he had everything he needed and would be leaving for New York that afternoon. I looked at the canvas. Lines and brush paths were everywhere, with blotches of many paint colors in no systematic pattern. Nothing I looked at had any resemblance of the actual work I had

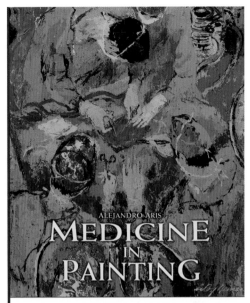

Cover of the medical art book.

been doing all week. How had I failed to convey the beautiful artistry of surgery to the master of the paint brush? I was deeply disappointed, but I did not let on to LeRoy. I thanked him and said goodbye. His final words were, "I'll call you Ted when I have something to show you." In the back of my mind, that could be twenty years away.

But it was not twenty years, it was only six weeks. He called to say the painting was done, and asked when I could come to his studio in New York to see it. I left on Friday night and was greeted by his assistant at 11 a.m. on Saturday. She ushered me to the floor above his very large studio. LeRoy graciously gave me a tour, showing some of his recently completed works and some of his early favorites. As we ended the tour he took me into an adjacent room where a painting on an easel was draped. He motioned me to come close and invited me to unveil his work. I did so and stood entranced. How could that canvas I saw in the dome smeared with paint blotches been transformed into this magnificent creation? It was done by a master. I felt humbled that he had captured the heart of our work so magnificently, and he knew I was thrilled.

"Ted, what do you want to name it?"

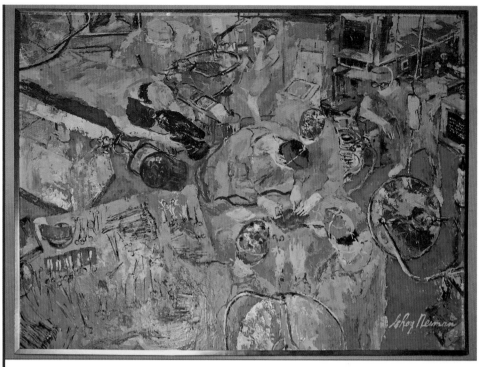

LeRoy Neiman's *Open Heart Surgery* hangs above the desk in my home study today.

"LeRoy, there could be only one name, *Open Heart Surgery*." LeRoy and I continued our friendship and always went out to dinner when I was in New York City. My YPO appearances dwindled over time.

Suddenly around 2002, a package arrived in my office. Upon opening it, there was an art book entitled *Medicine in Painting* and on the cover was the LeRoy painting *Open Heart Surgery* from 1982. The art book was assembled and written by Dr. Alejandro Aris, a heart surgeon from Barcelona, and Valentin Fuster, the famous cardiologist from NYC.

As I write this chapter so many years later, *Open Heart Surgery* hangs on the wall above my desk. The light coming through the window across the desert floor makes the colors even more vivid. I peer up and can see the operating team in motion, hands moving in synchrony. I can name each of its members and the covered patient beneath the drape. And I remember how I felt like a conductor overseeing a symphonic orchestra.

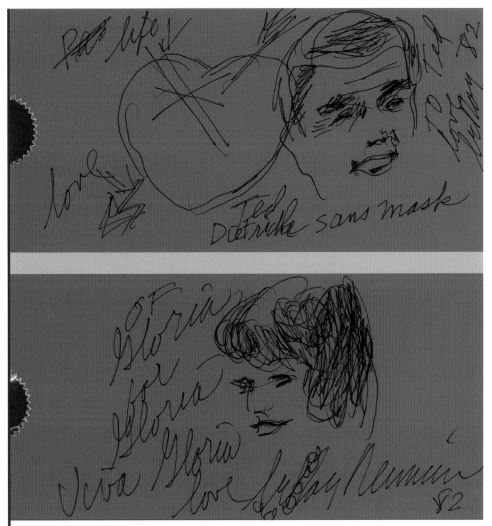

In February 1982, LeRoy sent Valentines cards to Gloria and me. It reminded me of the artistic progression of the finished product *Open Heart Surgery*. LeRoy was not only a great artist, but also a wonderful friend. He died in June 2012 at the age of ninety-one.

32

A Heart Surgeon on the Sidelines

There was a message on my desk to call, at my convenience, Bud Grant. I knew he was the head coach of the Minnesota Vikings football team, but I had no idea why he wanted to talk to me.

When I returned his call that afternoon, Bud said he was aware of the talks I was giving to the Young Presidents Organization, and he wanted to invite me to speak to the Viking's football team during their training camp in Minnesota. I questioned why these young super athletes would be interested in my talk, but then he volunteered that the players would be curious about the risk factors for heart and blood vessel disease, just like the presidents of many major corporations. I agreed.

Before I knew it, it was summer, and I was standing before the team. I have to confess, I was much more anxious there than when speaking before the presidents. I actually gave a similar presentation but included some football action. The event was amazingly successful and generated a lot of one-on-one communication with the players.

In hindsight, it would have been a great place to sell copies of my book, *Code Arrest: A Heart Stops*, written in 1974 with all of its information about heart disease prevention. Today, there seems to be even more interest in players' health after leaving football, a subject I alluded to while addressing them. The organization was very gracious. The experience gave me a new insight into professional football and how the sport can cause health issues in players' lives even years after leaving the sport.

As I became involved with NFL coaches and players, I learned that there were many parallels between their profession and mine. Obviously, both professions focus on health and physical fitness, both require coordinated teamwork, and we even share much of the same terminology. Each job is exciting and requires a high degree of discipline, and such considerations as sales, marketing, and business management are also mutually important.

In fact, it was the inauguration of an exciting football career experience. Within a few days, George Allen of the Washington Redskins contacted me, saying he had heard of the Vikings talk and wanted me to speak to his team.

That was the beginning of a long friendship with George. He called me at least once a week to talk about one thing or another and was always concerned about being healthy. (He ran every day but frequently ate ice cream sundaes.) He would invite me to the sidelines when I was in town or even for away games, and as a result I met many of the NFL personnel. The Commissioner, Pete Rozell, even went through our cardiovascular screening program at the Institute.

In 1981, the NFL funded a research project that was conducted by our Foundation. "Papa Bear" George Halas, owner of the Chicago Bears, presented the check to me personally at a Bears game in Chicago. This was the ultimate example of how I could meld two of my great loves—medicine and sports.

I could have ended it there and been ecstatic with the experience. However, George Allen was having some difficulty with his coaching

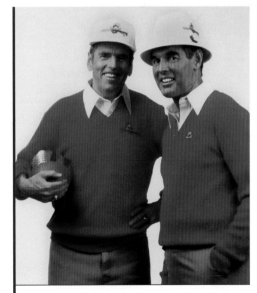

Coach Allen and me when we became the Arizona Wranglers.

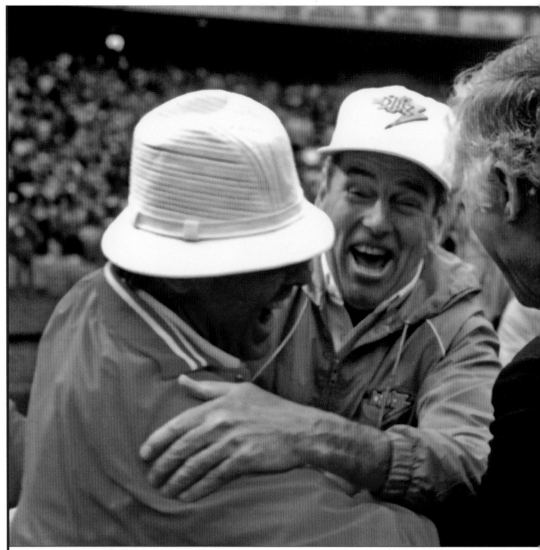

Coach Allen, Bill Harris (co-owner), and me after a Blitz victory in Chicago; this was the
first televised game of the USFL as well as its first touchdown!

contracts and entered a phase without a coaching position on an NFL team. Soon
enough, I got another call.

"Ted, there is interest in starting a new league. The United States Football
League, the USFL. Would you be interested in the Chicago Franchise?"

I had just sold my imaging company, ADR, so I knew I could invest even though
it seemed high risk. I met with George and his partner Bill Harris, and eventually

we became the owners of the Chicago Blitz in the new USFL. That was an entirely different life for me.

My son, Tad, also became involved, and the entire family was invested in enjoying this adventure. However, the trips between Phoenix and Chicago became difficult; it took too much time away from my medical practice. I was able to trade the

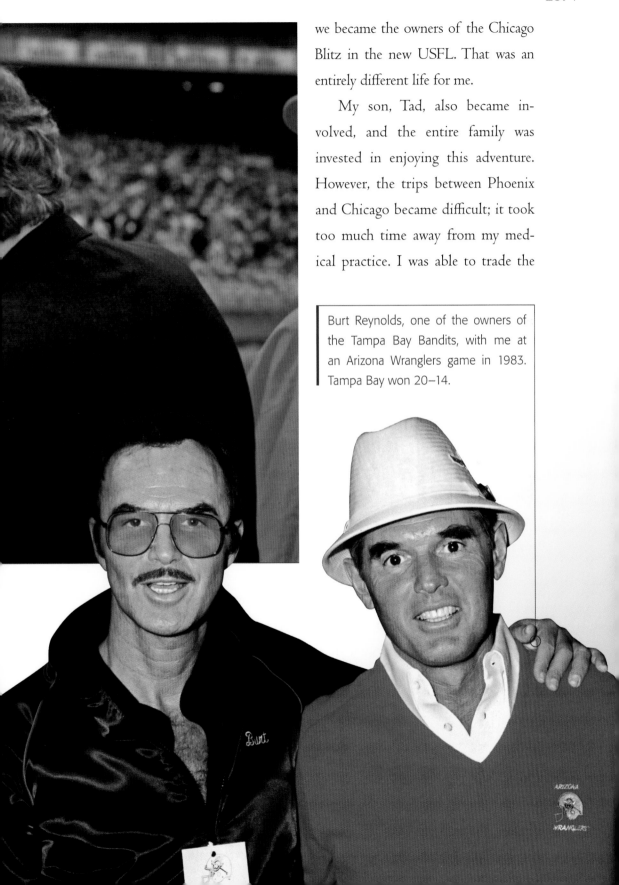

Burt Reynolds, one of the owners of the Tampa Bay Bandits, with me at an Arizona Wranglers game in 1983. Tampa Bay won 20–14.

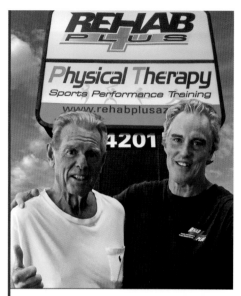

Warren Anderson and me in front of Rehab Plus.

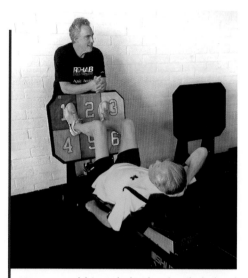

Warren and his Rehab Plus family helped me to overcome adverse effects of wearing heavy lead aprons for forty years.

Chicago Blitz franchise for the Arizona Wranglers and we made the move in the middle of the night.

It turned out to be a highlight for the AHI family. Most of the staff went to the games, and after each victory the lobby of the building was packed with celebrating AHI staff! George took the team to the initial championship game in Philadelphia, which we unfortunately lost. Ultimately about two years later, I sold my interest in order to initiate new programs for the Heart Institute. I would never have substituted that experience for anything.

I had a little part in building another great team.

Coach Allen was enthusiastic about strengthening exercises, and the football team hired Warren Anderson to fill this position and various other assignments. Over the years I lost track of Warren but he resurfaced recently when I needed some physical therapy related to all these years that I've worn the heavy lead aprons in the operating room to protect against radiation exposure. Warren was eager to establish a program for me, and we filmed a piece on radiation safety at his facility. I was pleased Warren agreed to be in the film along with his great facility and staff.

33

White Out

The year was 1985. We had seen more than satisfactory results with our cardiac transplantation program, and began to encounter patients who were candidates for heart and lung transplantation. This was familiar to me, due to the work on the heart-lung preservation chamber at Baylor. In fact many of the technical aspects were very similar.

One of the patients in particular turned out to be a special challenge. Peni Toni was a young forty-two-year-old teacher from California with pulmonary hypertension and congestive heart failure. She was very sick, and we delayed her operation for some time in hopes of reducing her operative risk. The actual operation went extremely well, and on the first postoperative day she was stable and alert on the ventilator.

I was very pleased, until I saw the early morning chest x-ray on the view box next to her bed. The entire right side of her chest film was completely white, otherwise known as a white out.

I immediately ordered up the bronchoscopy equipment and looked

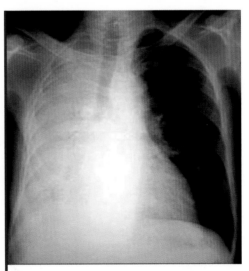

White out of the right lung, indicating no lung function.

down the trachea, but it was completely clear. I moved on to the bifurcation into the right and left main stem bronchi. I anticipated finding a blockage on the right, but it was as clear and open as the partner on the left. I obviously had the wrong diagnosis. There was no mucus plug, and no technical problem with the suturing.

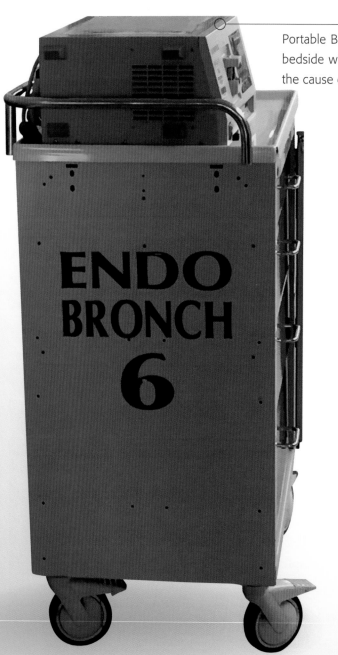

Portable Bronchoscope used at the bedside with Peni Toni to diagnose the cause of "white out."

I couldn't entertain any thought of weaning Peni from the respirator; she would have died within hours.

Fortunately, The Society of Thoracic Surgeons was holding a meeting at a hotel downtown. These were the leading heart and lung experts in the world. They would be able to help me with this terrible dilemma. I grabbed the x-ray, jumped into my car, and rushed toward the hotel. I wasn't sure what I would accomplish, but I had never experienced the white out phenomenon before without an explanation of the etiology. I knew many members present at the meeting, and one-by-one I asked for opinions on both the diagnosis and what to do. An hour later I left the hotel, really depressed. No one had any answers, and even worse, they did not seem interested in my problem or Peni's problem. But now, what to do?

Back at the hospital I went to her bedside and replaced the x-ray on the view box. Looking back and forth between Peni and the chest films, it occurred to me that Peni was a very small lady, or at least her chest was small. The donor was a male with normal heart and lungs. The problem became crystal clear: The lung on the right was too large for Peni's chest cavity. It was being compressed and as a result it could not expand. The result was a white out! (Not to be confused with the "white out" that occurred at the Penn State versus Michigan game on November 21, 2015, when all the Penn State fans wore white shirts.)

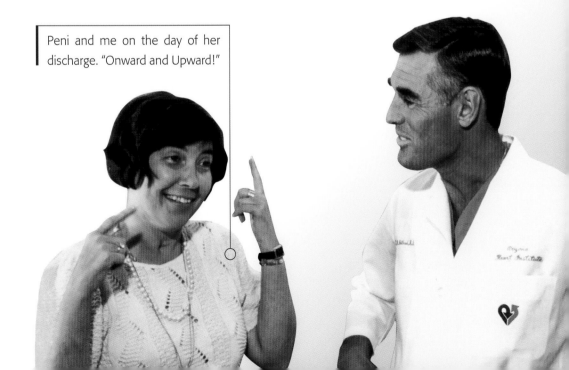

Peni and me on the day of her discharge. "Onward and Upward!"

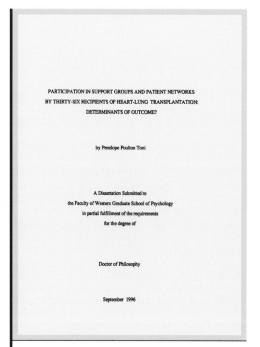

PARTICIPATION IN SUPPORT GROUPS AND PATIENT NETWORKS
BY THIRTY-SIX RECIPIENTS OF HEART-LUNG TRANSPLANTATION:
DETERMINANTS OF OUTCOME?

by Penelope Poulton Toni

A Dissertation Submitted to
the Faculty of Western Graduate School of Psychology
in partial fulfillment of the requirements
for the degree of

Doctor of Philosophy

September 1996

Peni Toni's PhD Thesis in 1996, eleven years after her transplant.

I am hard pressed to recall a time in my entire medical career when I felt more alone. My high-powered colleagues at the hotel were no help. There were no articles or textbooks that could guide me. I went back to Peni's bedside. She had the breathing tube in place that prevented her from talking, but her mind was pretty clear. So I explained the situation to her.

"The heart is working perfectly. The left lung is just fine, but we have a problem on the right. The donor lung is too large and won't function properly. I need to perform a little operation to remove a portion of that right lung and allow it to expand. You will be just fine!" How could I even tell her what the end result would be? I was not sure this had ever been done before.

Within the hour we were in the operating room. On opening the chest it was obvious that the right lung was too large. I removed the lower lobe. The remainder of the lung expanded, filled with fresh oxygen, and immediately took on the healthy pink color of well-oxygenated tissue. I took a deep breath. There had not been many times in my operating experience when I took a metabolic pause and said, "Thanks, God." Someone had to be shepherding me through this adventure and as a result Peni survived.

In preparation for this chapter, I contacted Peni. After her recovery she returned to California where the Stanford transplantation team managed her medication and further rehabilitation. She informed me that she had returned to school and ultimately received her Doctorate degree. She has had no rejection issues, and while the drugs are a little tough, she accepts that she will always

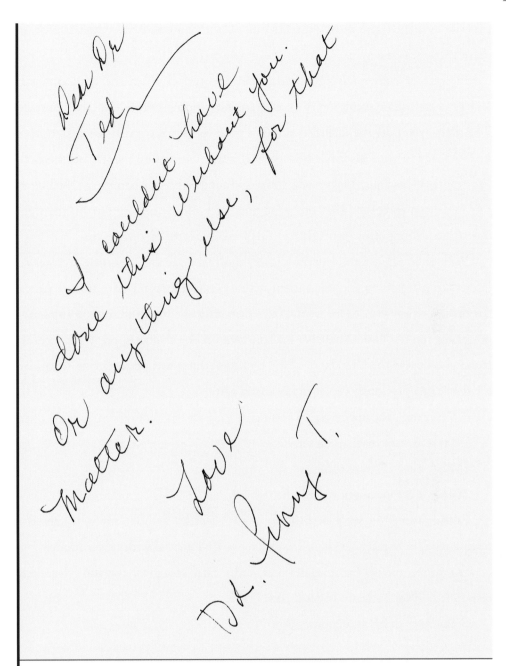

Dear Dr Ted —

I couldn't have done this without you. Or anything else, for that matter.

Love,

Dr. Penny T.

Note from Peni to me when she sent me her thesis book.

require them. She also revealed that she has outlived all of her transplant pals at Stanford. To my knowledge she is the longest living patient with a heart-lung transplant in the United States and perhaps the world (thirty years). I can assure you she is one of the most grateful out of the thousands of patients over all these years.

In spite of some early problems, if anyone ever doubted the value of heart and lung transplantation, Peni's case is an outstanding example to the contrary. The thank-you note she included is found in my personal copy of her dissertation in 1996, eleven years after her transplant. I remember before she left our hospital she expressed gratitude for her new heart and lungs with one comment: "Whoever they belonged to before, they are mine now, including a smaller one on the right due to the white out. It seems that is a legitimate degree of ownership."

Peni Toni's long-term survival is certainly spectacular. Recently, I received information regarding another patient with a positive long-term follow-up. At the conclusion of my visit to my dental hygienist, after she took the suction apparatus out of my mouth, I asked how her husband was feeling. "Oh just great. He recently had a checkup at the Cleveland Clinic and everything was perfect." She reminded me that I had previously replaced his aortic valve.

"When was that operation?" I inquired.

"It is now over twenty years ago."

"What kind of valve did I use, do you remember?"

"It was a bovine aortic valve." she replied.

Enthusiastically I suggested that over two decades without any problems is a terrific result. "Sometimes these valves have to be replaced with newer models."

She patted me on the shoulder and said, "He had a great surgeon!" I quickly responded, "No, I selected a good cow!"

Sometimes in life it all comes down to the luck of the draw.

34

King Hussein

Not surprisingly, I met many interesting people, some of them surgeons from around the world, while working with both Drs. DeBakey and Cooley.

One in particular was Dr. David Hanania. He was a cardiovascular surgeon from Amman, Jordan, who spent time in Houston while I was on the faculty. David and I became friends, and we kept in touch when he returned to Jordan. He was a general in the military and a close confidant of King Hussein.

David was in the process of establishing the King Hussein Medical Center and would frequently contact me with questions about his practice and even sent nurses and technicians to AHI for training.

In 1974, as the time for the inauguration of the King Hussein Medical Center drew near, David called and asked if I would participate and perform the first operation in the medical center. I accepted the invitation, obviously honored.

At about the same time, a local businessman by the name of Harold Minor heard about the plan in Amman. He had extensive relationships with the most influential families in Saudi Arabia and felt those connections might be helpful to the Arizona Heart Foundation. He approached me with the idea of joining the

A young King Hussein who presented his award to me while in Jordan.

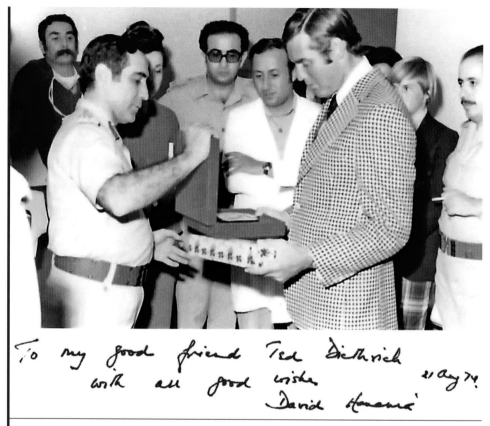

To my good friend Ted Diethrich with all good wishes   21 Aug 74.   David Hanania

Dr. David Hanania explaining to me the King Hussein Award after operating at the King Hussein Medical Center in Amman, Jordan. My son, Tad, is in the back row directly behind me.

Amman visit and touring some of the major cardiovascular centers in Saudi Arabia. This sounded like an exceptional opportunity. The plans were made, and I thought it would be great to have my young son, Tad, travel with me in that part of the world. It would be a new experience for both of us.

Jeddah, Saudi Arabia, was our first stop, followed by Riyadh, where I found myself extremely busy. Somehow the word had gotten out about my visit. In addition to visiting hospitals, arrangements were set up for me to do consultations on patients with a variety of cardiac and vascular diseases. It turned out to be a mixed bag of pathology; some heart, some blood vessel and some of both.

I had an assigned driver with instructions of where to take me, and there was an electrocardiogram technician and a small portable ECG machine to accompany me wherever I went. I saw some pretty bizarre ECG strips, maybe because the ECG leads were placed incorrectly by the technician. However, I did not make any unique diagnoses based on this particular information. There were so many visits, and so many patients; it became difficult to recall them all. However, there were two occasions that were exceptional—one social and one medical.

My major visit was at the military hospital where the head surgeon, a general, greeted me with a salute and open arms. Following a tour of the facilities, he had arranged a luncheon at his home with some colleagues, their wives, and business folks. We were taken into a large sitting room where the servants were offering tea and some sort of juices. After the usual introductions, the general asked if I wanted a drink since I had passed on the coffee. Before I even responded he took a couple of steps toward the wall, and opened two sliding panels displaying almost every kind of liquor imaginable. I knew this was against their religion, and it would have been very impolite to accept even if I had desired, so I offered a polite, "No, thank you."

There were two aspects of the Saudi Arabia visit that interested me the most. The medical aspect was pretty clear, but at the time the culture was somewhat confusing, such as the drinking of alcohol. After the offer of alcohol, my host directed me to folding doors that led out to a very large green grass yard. Stepping out, it was the first time it had dawned on me that there were no women in the first room. Outside, they were all seated at a long table on one side of the yard. Another similar table was near the opposite side, I presumed for the male guests.

"Doctor, where would you like to sit?" asked the head surgeon. Quickly thinking of my second mission to understand more about the culture, I replied, "Maybe with the ladies to broaden my education on your culture."

He ushered me to a seat in the middle of the ladies' table where all had their faces covered. He introduced me to the lady on either side, and I smiled and let them know how nice it was to meet them. Both were extremely friendly, spoke English well, and seemed eager to talk about any subject I brought up, from schools to recreation to vacations. I stayed away from politics. As lunch progressed and the ladies and I began to know each other better, conversations flowed like it was a U.S. picnic. Finally, I could not refrain any longer. I had to refer to the seating of the men and women separately. They responded with the answer I expected: "It's the custom."

My next question was obvious, "If you don't get together, how do you learn about each other?" The lady on my right was quick to respond.

"We all have our own personal chauffeur. If we pause at a stoplight and see a handsome man in the car next to ours we just...(she took her right hand and gradually pulled her veil to expose a pretty smile). "It works well, and who knows how it will end up?" I felt that I shouldn't bring it up anymore and changed the subject immediately but became much more observant at the street corners.

Most of the requested consultations resulted in my driver taking me to a residence, which usually was a large palace of a royal family member. It seemed everyone were members of the royal family. While I was still not clear on who was a king and who a prince, one night I was deposited at the palace of the oldest living monarch in Saudi Arabia.

By this time I was used to the sizes of the dwellings; however, on being led through the monarch's door I thought I was on a football field. The only difference was the lack of grass. Instead, there was the most expansive, widest, and beautiful

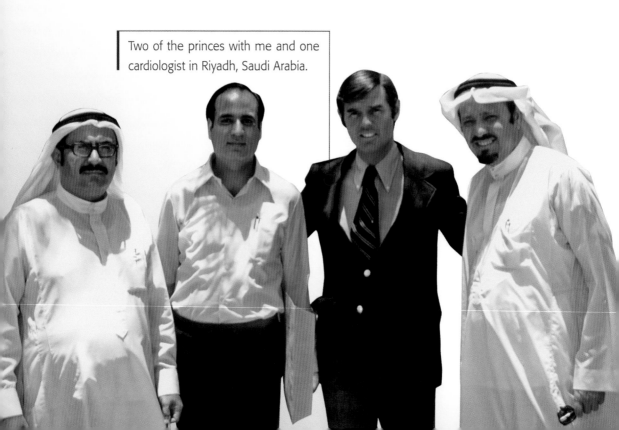

Two of the princes with me and one cardiologist in Riyadh, Saudi Arabia.

oriental carpets I had ever seen, extending before me from the door to a large throne-like chair where the oldest-living monarch sat.

Two younger princes escorted me down the carpet until I finally stood at the foot of the giant chair. Indeed, he looked like the oldest of something. He was pale and obviously weak, but still sitting up. I spoke to my accompanying princes, who seemed to understand me quite well. I suggested that in order to examine the monarch I would need to have him in bed. They hurriedly removed him from the chair and brought him into a bedroom annexed to the great hall.

When I saw all the medicines lined up near the bed stand, it was clear that he had been under the care of a physician. The ECG technician took a tracing: old infarction, significant bradycardia. His blood pressure was off the charts, 210/110. Auscultation of the lungs produced the expected; he was suffering from pulmonary edema. A quick look at the ankles confirmed the fluid overload. The heart was enlarged with distant sounds. His breathing seemed labored. I immediately told the prince to elevate the monarch to a more erect position.

I began to look at the medicines and saw digitalis, a diuretic, and anti-hypertensive medication. Interestingly, no matter where you are in the world, drugs for the heart are very much the same. I turned to the prince holding the vials.

"Does he take all these medications on a regular basis?"

In perfect English the prince responded, "He does not like to take medications and often refuses the pills." I was shocked, not by the answer but by the perfect English.

"Where did you go to school?" I asked.

"I took my graduate education at the University of Arizona in Tucson, Arizona," he replied.

What a small world. I was thousands of miles from my home in Phoenix, and this young prince was educated at a college two hours from there. And now there I was in Saudi Arabia, consulting on his desperately ill relative.

I instructed the prince that he must personally be responsible for the medication. It was no wonder the old fellow had blood pressures off the charts. Beyond these instructions, there was not much I could do. The monarch did not have much longer in the world, and the best I could do was excuse myself and leave the palace. At the very least, I did not want to be seen as a contributor to his demise. It was just like the scenario with Dr. Kahn and the heat exchanger in the emergency unit years before. I have never been averse to treating a high-risk patient, but this was obviously hopeless.

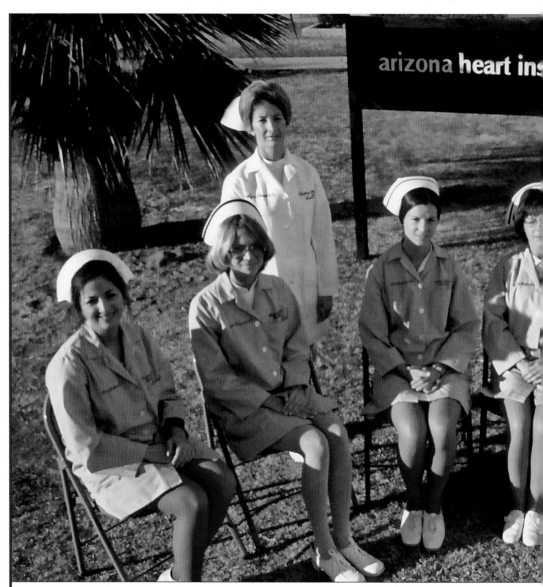

Cardiovascular Nurse Specialist class of 1975 with Carolyn House as instructor. On the far right is student Abla Dababeneh, RN from Amman, Jordan, sent by Dr. David Hanania for training in preparation of the opening of the King Hussein Medical Center.

It wasn't so bad being directed from one consultation to another, but there was one thing I definitely did not expect. This was the orchestrated event at the end of the trip. Some of the medical doctors caring for the patients were preparing a list of those they considered good candidates for my care in Amman, Jordan, the next stop on the journey. On the last day there was a fairly large gathering of medical people in the

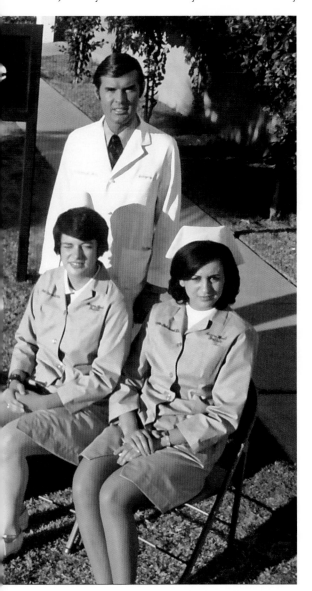

hotel lobby. This was to be a farewell, but it turned out to be the presentation of a patient list to accompany us on a military C-130 plane to Amman. These doctors had been so hospitable and gracious that I had no option but to board the transport plane and strap in for the flight.

This was definitely not first-class on Emirates Airlines but rather a very basic army transport plane with a group of patients that I did not recognize. More important, I had little idea of their medical conditions. A couple of physicians joined this flying party, which was helpful because during the entire flight I moved from seat to seat to interview each patient with the accompanying doctor interpreting.

By the time we landed in Amman, I had made complete rounds and had a patient list. The spellings of their names were mostly unreadable, but next to each name I made an indication of what the patient would require. It was a wide variety of diagnoses. However, the most important aspect

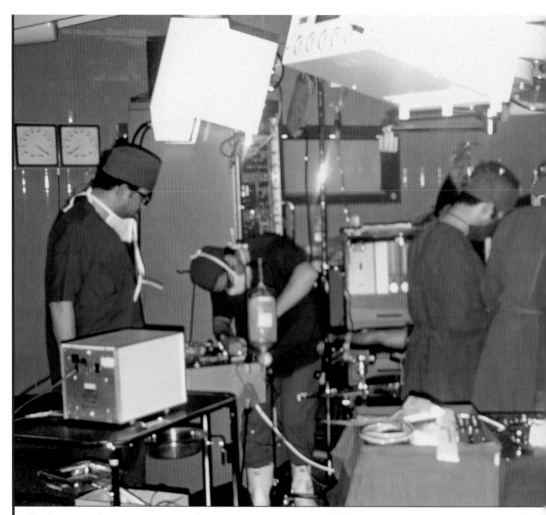

The first open heart operation in the new King Hussein Medical Center in Amman, Jordan was performed in the mid-1970s.

was that the suspected diagnosis determined exactly what care we might be able to provide.

I made a fundamental category list based upon what information I had without further testing: "Should be easy, uncertain, and no way!" The latter category included patients who should not have been on the flight; these patients were too ill and would require complicated procedures for which we had not planned. Of course, I would reserve the final decision until I reviewed the list with David Hanania in Amman.

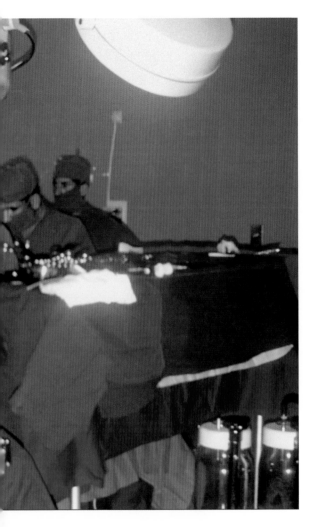

To this day I do not know how the whole transportation from Saudi Arabia to Jordon was orchestrated. Clearly it had to have David and King Hussein's endorsement.

David had done an excellent job organizing the new King Hussein Medical Center. We all enjoyed working together and the results were excellent, probably due to our careful patient selection.

In addition to operating on this trip, I also taught and gave lectures. One day we were having lunch with some of the staff and King Hussein, and near the end he asked what I would enjoy seeing in his country. I replied that I had read and heard so much about the Golan Heights; it would be nice to see that area first hand. The next day upon leaving the palace, we were directed to cars waiting to transport us to the military helicopter pads. Within minutes, we were headed to the Golan Heights.

Our military guide was eager to help us explore not only the geography of the area we were observing but also the history. Obviously, that history was skewed positively for the Palestinians and negatively for the Israelis. As I watch the world news today, it is apparent that some forty years later, not much has changed in their attitudes about the situation.

While having dinner that evening with David he gave me his Palestinian perspective and family story, which was actually very emotional. It was fair to say at

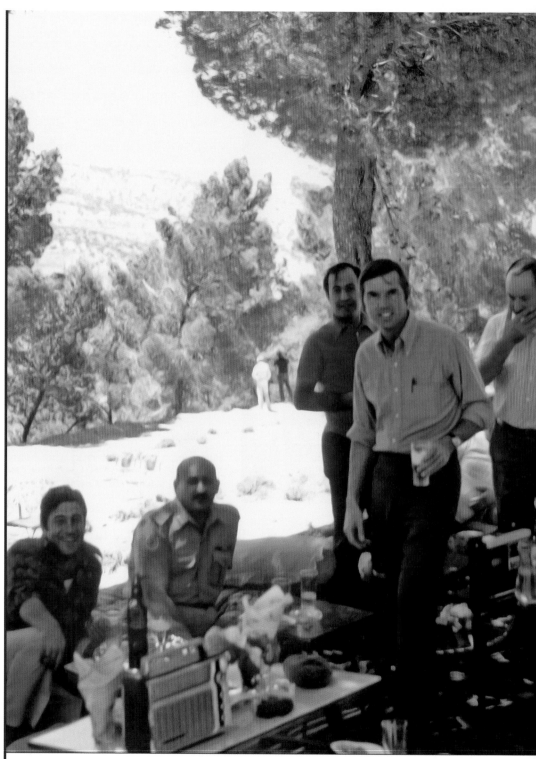

A peaceful picnic with the Jordanian team on the edge of the Golan Heights.

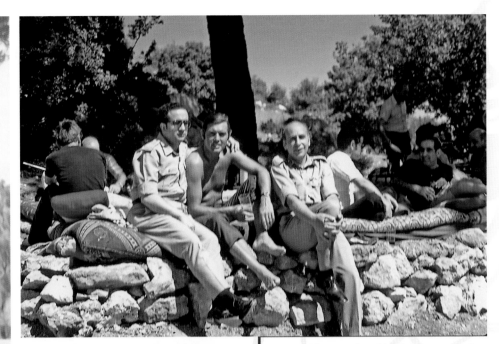

Dr. David Hanania with his arm around me while at the picnic.

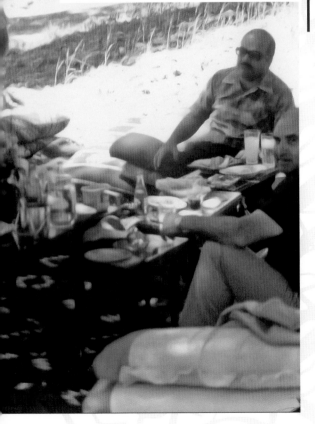

that moment I was a sympathizer for his position. Several years later I traveled to Israel with my friend Marty Kaplitt and heard an equally compelling but different side of the story. One wonders if it will ever be resolved.

The trip ended in Beirut, Lebanon, with a wonderful party given in my honor. Peter Jennings was present, and when I spoke to him about the visit to the Golan Heights, he convinced me to keep an even, balanced position. Good advice, even today.

That was not the end of the Amman connection. I returned on many occasions and operated on several people, including relatives of the King. During one visit there was a birthday party for the Queen, which was a special affair.

During the fall of 2012, David asked for my opinion on a patient from Chad, North Africa, who contacted him for advice on a thoracic aneurysm. David sent the CT images to the Institute. Some physicians in Paris were advocating an operation that would involve the entire aortic arch but potentially resulting in major complications. I suggested to David the patient go to Modena, Italy, where we could use a device being developed by Cardiatis, a Belgium company. That plan was set into motion. Unfortunately, the aneurysm was not completely sealed and an additional graft would be needed. I made arrangements for Dr. Sherif Sultan from Ireland to perform the surgery at David's facility. I was not available to travel. Another example of how colleagues around the world can work cooperatively together.

This multilayer flow modulator (MFM) causes the aneurysm to thrombose, while maintaining blood flow to major organs and structures.

35

Bordeaux Red Wine

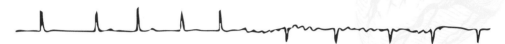

I was in Bordeaux, France, at a vascular surgical meeting in 1992. The enthusiasm for these new procedures was escalating, and many of my friends, from Europe and beyond, were present. At a small gathering on the last evening, a few of us were in the bar relaxing and reflecting on all that we had learned. As more wine was poured, the conversation was directed to another topic.

"Ted, there is a need for a new society that represents the exciting material presented here…an endovascular society."

This was from Professor Takis Balas, a longtime friend. He is a famous Greek vascular surgeon and was the President of the European Society for Vascular Surgery in 1994. He was well known for his abilities to create societies. They were directing this comment to me, since I had become identified as a kind of leader of the band, the one that was playing endovascular music around the world. But the last thing in the world that I thought any of us needed was one more society. We were already saturated with societies of all kinds.

Suddenly, someone suggested that a new endovascular society could be the impetus for a new journal devoted to these evolving endovascular techniques. It did not take another glass of Bordeaux to whet my appetite for that suggestion. It was exactly what we needed: a peer-reviewed journal with an international editorial board that was capable of communicating our scientific mission to the surgical community, and perhaps beyond.

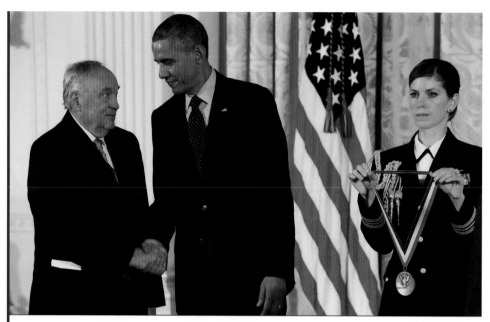

Tom Fogarty receiving an award from President Obama.

Before the evening was over, this self-appointed group had elected me as president of the International Society for Endovascular Surgery (ISES) and editor of its new journal, tentatively named the *Journal of Endovascular Surgery*. My first recommendation was to name the famous inventor, Thomas Fogarty, MD as co-editor-in-chief of the journal. This turned out to be a special nomination because in November 2014, Tom Fogarty's pursuits were recognized when President Obama presented him with the National Medal of Technology and Innovation. A recognition whole-heartedly supported by the ISES membership.

My Bordeaux colleagues also gave me the assignment of putting the society and the journal together legally and launching a membership drive. Fortunately for me, I had just the person to handle this.

Many years prior, when we had just moved to the new Arizona Heart Institute, I had been thinking of hiring a writer to work with me and Video Arts Studio on our many projects. One day, my administrative assistant, Bet Levander, caught me between cases. She said a young lady whom I should meet was in the AHI lobby. "She may have some of the skill sets that you have been looking for."

As I descended the long stairway leading from the second level down to the main floor, my eyes connected to a very attractive young lady on the couch at the far end of the lobby. I introduced myself and she replied "Nice to meet you Doctor, I am Rebecca Bowman." The interview far exceeded my allotted time, but I immediately knew I had a special talent in my presence. I asked to be excused to attend to a matter upstairs. There was no other matter. I wanted to see Bet and have her hire Rebecca on the spot. I did not even want her to leave the building without confidence that she was needed here and had a job. Bet as usual closed the deal, and I went back downstairs to welcome Rebecca to the AHI team.

That was thirty-seven years ago. Rebecca made enormous contributions to our program and to the Society, but perhaps her twenty-year leadership as executive editor of the *Journal of Endovascular Therapy* stands at the top of the list. In 2014, the

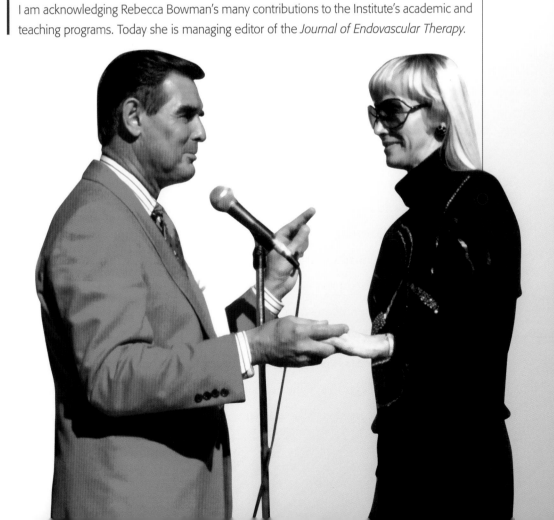

I am acknowledging Rebecca Bowman's many contributions to the Institute's academic and teaching programs. Today she is managing editor of the *Journal of Endovascular Therapy.*

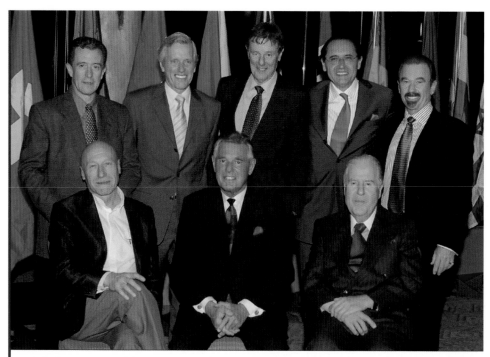

Original organizers of the International Society of Endovascular Specialists. Front row: Patrice Bergeron, MD; me; and Panagiotis E. Balas, MD. Back row: Frank J. Criado, MD; Jacques Bleyn, MD; Alan E. Bray, MD; Jacques Busquet, MD; and Rodney A. White, MD.

JEVT became the highest ranked journal in the world devoted to peripheral vascular interventions. In all of these years and numerous projects, she has never failed me or her colleagues. Bet had found a jewel.

Sometimes bad things happen when a group of young vascular surgeons drink too much red wine. Thankfully, that night in Bordeaux when we founded the ISES was not one of those times. History will show that the decisions emanating from the bar that evening made a major impact on the future of vascular surgery around the world.

At the time, the emphasis on "surgeons" and "surgery" seemed obvious—that was who we were and what we did. However, as time passed, I became convinced the endovascular evolution was not going to be successful if it only emphasized surgeons. The field was much larger, compelled to have multiple disciplines involved—surgeons, radiologists, cardiologists, vascular medicine specialists and no doubt, many others.

I do not want to make it seem that I was the Lone Ranger in espousing this philosophy, but among many of my vascular surgical colleagues, I indeed turned out to be a loner.

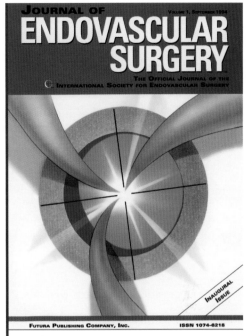

The first issue of *JEVS*.

Because of my position as president of the ISES and co-editor of the journal with Dr. Fogarty, I made an executive decision. I guess today it would be parallel to President Obama's "I have a phone, I have a pen" comment. Indeed, I was definitely not that arrogant, but very determined. The name had to be changed to reflect the future direction.

Thus, in 2000, the *Journal of Endovascular Surgery* became the *Journal of Endovascular Therapy* (*JEVT*) and the International Society for Endovascular Surgery became the International Society of Endovascular Specialists (ISES).

Was this move well received? No!

"You sold us out!" shouted the surgeons. "You're no better than Benedict Arnold!"

Indeed, it took some rehabilitation on my part to bring the folks around, but there was no doubt in my mind about the wisdom of these decisions. The current success of the *JEVT* alone attests to that conclusion.

As the endovascular society was growing and gaining membership, the Society for Vascular Surgery (SVS) board initiated some reorganization under the initiative of Dr. Robert Hobson, including one that directly affected ISES. SVS changed its membership rules, permitting more surgeons to join with broader potential to participate in the society's activities. Even more important, ISES was invited to have an active member on the SVS board with all the rights of the other board members. As president of ISES, I was appointed to the SVS board. That may not appear to be a positive consequence, but in fact it was.

The SVS board was composed of mainly vascular surgeons, many representing university programs. I was representing another society, one that was at least subliminally promoting the use of balloons, lasers, stents, and minimizing the function of the scalpel. I would sit around the large conference table and promote our point of view, but the other members were not very interested in what I would say.

As I've said, I was a loner, but I could gradually see a slight shift in the pendulum. This was really apparent when a professor of vascular surgery from one of the major East Coast universities approached me during a coffee break and asked if it would be possible to send one of his residents to train with me. I knew then there was at least a small crack in the iceberg.

Other presidents of ISES were also subsequently appointed to the SVS board. Dr. Rodney White, Professor/Chief of Vascular Surgery at UCLA, one of the pioneers of the laser field, served a three-year term. At present, one of my first vascular fellows, Dr. Ali AbuRahma, Professor and Chief of Vascular Surgery at West Virginia University, serves on behalf of the ISES.

In 2013, I had an invitation from Dr. James Yao to participate in a video production by SVS in regards to my endovascular work. In the video, a dozen or so surgeons were interviewed by colleagues like Dr. Roger Gregory, Dr. James Yao, and others to document much of the history of vascular surgery. Jimmy was very kind in providing a copy of the interview, and I used some of the content in this book *SLED*, which in itself is a history of the endovascular evolution.

At the end of the interview, Jimmy let the cat out of the bag: he told me I was being awarded the Medal for Innovation in Vascular Surgery at the annual SVS meeting in San Francisco.

I never expected a special award for what I did; that was simply how I had always operated. However,

Dr. Roger Gregory, key interviewer for the *Society of Vascular Surgery* history film.

I must confess that during President Peter Gloviczki's presentation, where I was awarded the Medal for Innovation in Vascular Surgery in front of the surgical society, I did not have dry eyes.

"Introduction of Edward B. Diethrich, MD, 2013 Recipient of the Medal for Innovation in Vascular Surgery," by Peter Gloviczki, MD, President, Society for Vascular Surgery, presented at the 2013 Vascular Annual Meeting of the Society for Vascular Surgery, San Francisco, California, May 30–June 3, 2013.

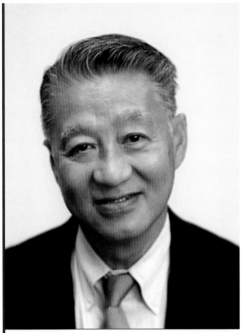

Dr. James Yao, strong supporter for the SVS award presented to me by Dr. Gloviczki.

"The SVS Medal for Innovation in Vascular Surgery was established in 2006 and since then it has been awarded to four distinguished, extremely talented pioneer vascular surgeons. This award is given to an individual or individuals whose contribution to vascular surgery has had a transforming impact on the practice or science of vascular surgery. This year I have the privilege of introducing the fifth recipient of this prestigious award.

He has had a distinguished career as an extraordinary vascular and cardiothoracic surgeon, leader, and innovator. The list of innovations attributed to him is long, starting in 1962 with invention of the sternal saw for opening the chest and continuing with his legacy of establishing and directing an internationally known Heart Foundation and Heart Institute.

He has been a pioneer; a mover and shaker in the endovascular revolution, and his contribution to surgical education has been legendary. He organized the first live telecast of open-heart surgery to an international audience. His annual endovascular meetings have attracted physicians from all corners of the world. The educational value of his presentations has been unique. The large number of live telecasts he includes in these meetings has contributed to better and faster training of hundreds of vascular specialists worldwide.

He developed one of the first ultrasound companies and contributed to the development of a preservation chamber for heart transplantation. His role in introducing one of the endovascular aortic grafts in the U.S. has been essential, and he is a founder and medical director of this device company. Over the past ten years alone, he was involved in founding three organizations dedicated to advancing the practice of vascular surgery. One develops and manufactures endoluminal grafts; the other is a Translational Research Center, dedicated to preclinical and clinical research in new and developing technologies. And more recently he started a corporation devoted to the prevention and management of cardiovascular disease, with an emphasis on non-traditional medicine. He is founder, Past President, and Chairman of the Board of the International Society of Endovascular Specialists.

Ladies and gentlemen, for his many contributions to innovation in endovascular surgery and for improving the education of generations of vascular surgeons and endovascular specialists, it is a distinct honor and privilege to present the 2013 SVS Medal of Innovation in Vascular Surgery to the Medical Director of the Arizona Heart Foundation and the Founder of the Arizona Heart Institute, Dr. Edward B. Diethrich."

The entire audience stood and applauded as the President presented me the award; it was a special moment in time. "Thank you, Dr. Gloviczki, for those kind words," I said as I accepted the award.

"Thank you, Peter, and thank you society members. I feel humbled by this award because as I look out into the audience, I can see many friends who have helped me and contributed greatly to whatever success I have had. We just heard a wonderful lecture about the innovation and advancement of technology over the past years. I was indeed involved in that evolution. I started seven or eight companies involved in various innovative approaches to diagnosis and treatment of cardiovascular disease. But I think the award you have presented to me today, which I very much appreciate, is not an award for me personally but rather an award for all of us who over the years have been working toward moving in a different direction. For a number of years, I was on the Board of the Vascular Society and I had to sit in the corner because people didn't like me very much. They would say, 'Who is that crazy Ted Diethrich who is out there trying to teach us some-thing about endovascular therapy?' Well fortunately, that all changed, and I believe the wonderful thing in accepting this award is that I am re-ally accepting it for all of us vascular

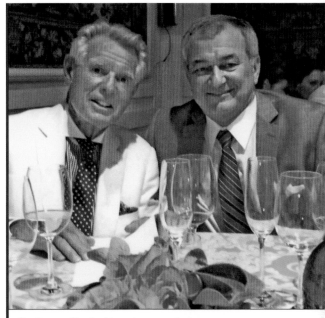

Dr. Peter Gloviczki and me at the restaurant Villa Trissino of the Marzotto family. It is located in Trissino, a small village in the Vicenza City area. It was June 28, 2012, during the meeting of Professor Deriu from Padova, Italy. We were discussing the future of vascular surgery.

surgeons, all of you and the society as a whole, because together we have moved forward in a very progressive way."

"We have together taken the new challenges of surgical transition into less invasive endovascular approaches for the future. I believe that is our future. I thank the society and the nominating committee."

All I could think about was the ride I had been on since I was the first ISES representative on the SVS Board for three years. It was a time when very few members would talk to me, believing that I was trying to sabotage vascular surgery. But there I was, at the annual meeting of SVS, where at least my colleagues appreciated my small contribution.

36

Athens

Hippocrates is frequently acknowledged as the "father" of Western Medicine. The Physician's Oath, to which his name is attributed but his authorship not verified, has been a component of our medical practice for decades.

Greek surgeons and physicians have taken a leading role, both in clinical and educational endeavors. One such contributor in the current era is Professor Takis Balas. As mentioned in the previous chapter, Takis was a founding member of the International Society for Endovascular Surgery as well as many others.

Over several years, Takis and I had a special arrangement where Greek patients would come to Phoenix for endovascular procedures. On one of these visits, Takis asked me to entertain the idea of performing live cases during the annual meeting of the European Society of Vascular Surgery, which was going to be held in Athens the year of his presidency. This European vascular community clearly had not accepted the endovascular approach I was espousing, and he felt it could be a significant contribution

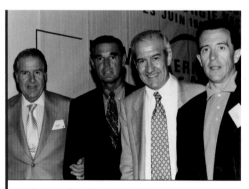

Left to right: Dr. Takis Balas, me, and Drs. Castelani and Creado at the workshop in Ajaceo, Corsica, for industrial leaders and physician researchers to discuss new devices and technologies to treat arterial and venous disease.

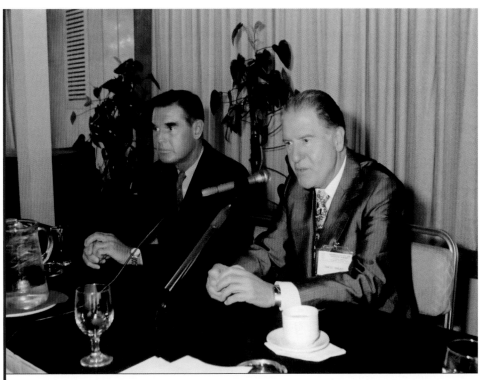

Dr. Balas and me at a press conference interview after the live case demonstration from Phoenix to Athens, Greece, at the time of the European Vascular Society Meeting. I never knew he was such a marketing expert.

to the meeting. After all, he pretty much controlled the program as the Society President. I, of course, was eager to accept the challenge, so the preparations were initiated.

The plan was to have Dick Williams of VAS travel to Athens and set everything up for the satellite transmission. I was to perform two or three interesting endovascular cases in Phoenix, and then quickly fly overnight to Athens in time to deliver a keynote lecture the next afternoon.

Takis felt that this telecast and lecture "double punch" would be a wakeup call for the society members who exhibited a European conservatism toward new endovascular explorations. The procedures went very well; however, I was a little disappointed in the lack of questions from the audience. Due to the uniqueness of the transmission, I guess I expected there to be a more active exchange of Q&A,

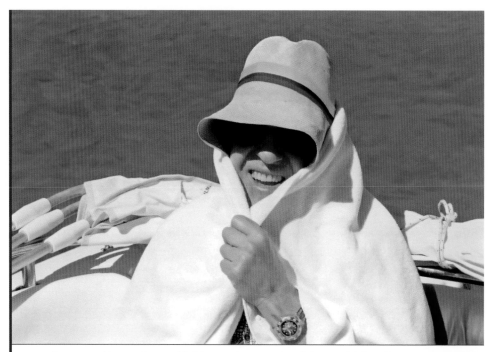

As serious as Takis was in establishing societies around the world, he also appreciated the lighter side of life as he had fun on the beach while at the workshop in Corsica.

both positive and negative. Takis was a great moderator, and that was helpful; he was also the loudest "clapper" when we concluded and signed off the live telecast. On my flight over I had already begun to wonder how I would be received the next afternoon in Athens, but I had many hours to ponder that concern.

Dick Williams greeted me at the hotel with a broad smile, indicating that, from his reconnaissance, the cases were well received. The auditorium was full, and I went directly to the podium for the lecture. Takis had assembled a panel of some of the most important European surgeons. After the forty-minute lecture, I would grade our exchange as friendly, but certainly not, "Well this young surgeon from the United States is going to change the vascular surgery world!"

I had never thought of Takis as a marketing expert, but that was a miscalculation on my part.

Over the next four days, Takis had booked me on the radio, several TV shows, and many newspaper interviews. What had I said to the ethics committee of the

Maricopa County Medical Society? "I am going to educate the public about cardiovascular disease." At the time, I did not appreciate it would be a worldwide effort.

As I was stepping down from the podium an older gentleman introduced himself as Professor Orthodoxos Papazoglou.

"Your presentation was beyond belief. Don't be disappointed if all these Brits don't jump on your bandwagon," he acknowledged. "I have a son just finishing his surgical training. Would there be a possibility for him to study a year or two with you?" So my mission was at least partially accomplished.

Eventually his son came to the AHI, the fellow that we would nick-

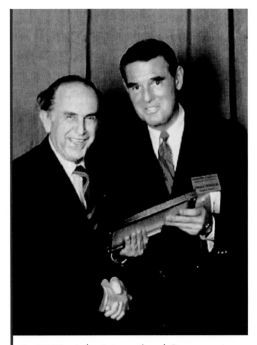

In 2002, at the International Congress, I presented Professor Orthodoxos Papazoglou with a membership certificate to the society. His son, Konstantinos Papazoglou later came to Phoenix to study with our team, making a significant contribution in endovascular grafting.

name Dr. Papa. He spent two years with us and was very helpful in developing our endovascular graft program.

Upon returning to Greece, he established an endovascular program in Thessaloniki and became a leader in the Greek vascular community.

Following the Athens trip, we normally would have two or more Greek patients referred to our service at AHI. On top of that, I continued to receive invitations to speak at many meetings in Europe. The endovascular evolution was sprouting roots.

37

Hot Tip Laser

Throughout all my world travels for business, one of the most frequent questions I am asked is how did I become involved, or more precisely, initiate endovascular therapy? This is a true example of how serendipity has flowed through my life.

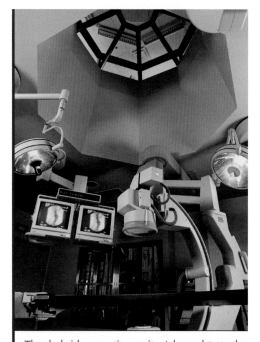

The hybrid operating suite I brought to the U.S. in 1971, complete with a radiolucent operating table, C-Arm angiographic unit, and seen here assembled in a special room with a dome for viewing the operation procedure.

Much of these you will remember from earlier in the book: A medical visit to Acapulco, where I was introduced to frontenis, followed by the building of the first frontenis court in the U.S.; playing in San Sebastian on the U.S. Olympic Frontenis Team; Dr. DeBakey's overbooked schedule, which placed me in the position to see Dr. Hans Moore of Philips Medical Systems. My persistence to have high-quality intraoperative angiography, and the first real hybrid operating room at the Arizona Heart Institute at St. Joseph's hospital. And then there was the Hot Tip Laser.

Once we had the Philips angiography equipment in the hybrid operating room, the potential to introduce new technologies for increasing blood flow and repairing arterial defects expanded greatly.

The Trimedyne Company in California developed a new laser technology to open blocked arteries. Dr. Rodney White from Harbor UCLA, who would later become president of the ISES, was working with them, and I visited him for some training. I was fascinated with the concept and began our own course at the Arizona Heart Institute.

INTERNATIONAL CONGRESS ON LASER APPLICATIONS IN VASCULAR SURGERY

FEBRUARY 14, 15, & 16, 1988
RED LION'S LA POSADA
RESORT HOTEL
SCOTTSDALE, ARIZONA

The first International Congress initiating lasers and laser application in vascular surgery; it was the inauguration of our annual February meeting which lasted twenty-six years.

It became so popular that our inaugural International Congress in 1988 revolved all around the topic of the laser. Many different types of lasers were developed, but the Hot Tip was the most popular. In the majority of patients we could open the arterial blockages in the lower extremity arteries and restore blood flow to the foot.

In time a variety of nuances were incorporated in the procedure. For example, a cardiologist from San Francisco stopped by his local Dunkin' Donuts store for a coffee. He observed the shiny frosting on some of the donuts. He had the idea that after the artery was opened with the laser, the hot tip could be rapidly passed up and down the artery, leaving a supposedly

Laser was one of the earliest techniques in endovascular surgery. The International Congress in 1988 was the introduction of a new era.

A glazed donut. Unfortunately the laser did not create any similar surface on the inner aspects of the arterial wall, but the concept created an interesting marketing hype for the company's product.

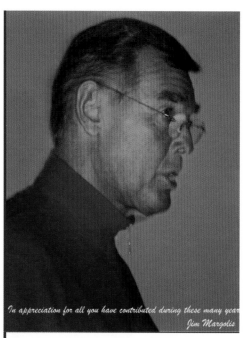

smoother inner surface. We nicknamed this procedure "glazing" and, indeed, the completed angiogram looked remarkably better. The problem was that the "glaze" was short lived, and a few months later the ugly irregularities had returned on the lining of the artery. Several months after the procedure, our studies showed the patency rate of the treated arteries was very low.

This taught me an important concept: working within the artery in a less invasive manner reduces the need for incisions, blood transfusions, and long rehabilitation. In the back of my mind, this was the beginning of an innovative concept for endovascular surgery and the beginning of a new treatment evolution.

Our laser conference to treat vascular disease created great interest among the vascular surgeons; however, one Miami cardiologist, Dr. James Margolis, joined me enthusiastically and began to promote the less invasive technologies to the cardiology community. He initiated his own annual conference in Snowmass, Colorado, incidentally where my family has a ski condominium. Jim invited me each February to participate, but when I looked around the auditorium I felt lonely. I was the only surgeon in attendance. Over the

In appreciation for all you have contributed during these many years
Jim Margolis

Gift from Jim Margolis.

years that changed, and our friendship was enhanced by a mutual passion for sport (snow skiing) and the endovascular treatment of vascular disease. He held his 30th annual meeting in 2015. I was not able to attend, the only one I ever missed, and he was so very kind to send me this picture showing his appreciation for my contributions over the years.

The most dramatic development in the endovascular field was the introduction of endografting to treat aneurysmal disease. It's not uncommon in the history of medicine that significant

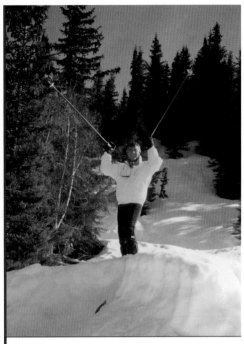

The Margolis meeting in Snowmass was a combination of work and great skiing.

contributors or scientific endeavors go unrecognized or are not attributed to the creator. This is the case of Professor Nikolay L. Volodos of the Ukraine.

I first met Professor Volodos in 1994 when he was an honored guest at the Arizona Heart Foundation's International Congress on Endovascular Interventions. I spoke with him briefly, but the language barrier prevented much scientific discussion. It was a missed opportunity that would not be set right until April 2012, when I sat transfixed at Roger Greenhalgh's Charing Cross Symposium in London listening to Professor Krassi Ivancev, a friend of Professor Volodos. Ivancev was head of the Complex Endovascular Treatment Team at the Royal Free Hospital in Hampstead, London and was delivering a talk on behalf of his Ukrainian colleague, who could not get a travel visa.

Professor Volodos' material was enormously impressive. At first blush, one might anticipate crude facilities with rudimentary engineering equipment. On the contrary, extensive multiyear preclinical studies incorporating flow models, physiological assessments, and animal implantations with subsequent detailed

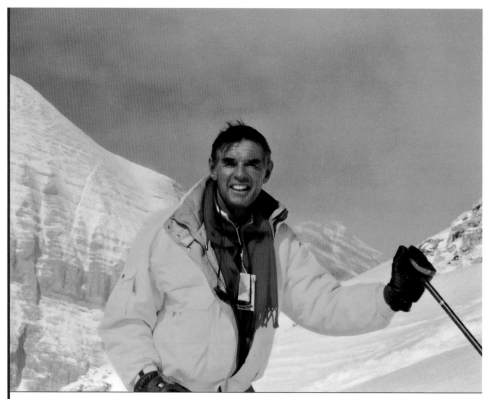

Cruising the big burn in Snowmass in between scientific sessions was no match for the exciting thrills of the challenges of the Dolomites in Italy.

histological analysis preceded the first clinical trials in patients with iliac, aortoiliac, thoracic, and abdominal aortic lesions. Indeed, I believe that our own FDA would respect the depth, breadth, and sophistication of the professor's laboratory and experimental methodology.

We honored many distinguished physicians from around the world at our annual International Congress meetings. My mentor, Dr. Denton Cooley, from Baylor College of Medicine, was awarded the Lifetime Achievement Award in 1995 during one of these meetings.

In 2012, at the 26th annual iCON meeting in Phoenix, we honored Professor Volodos and prepared a supplement of the *Journal of Endovascular Therapy* entitled *Historical Perspective—Endovascular Aneurysm Repair: Stent-Graft Development Behind the Iron Curtain. A Tribute to Ukrainian Surgeon Dr. Nikolay L. Volodos.*

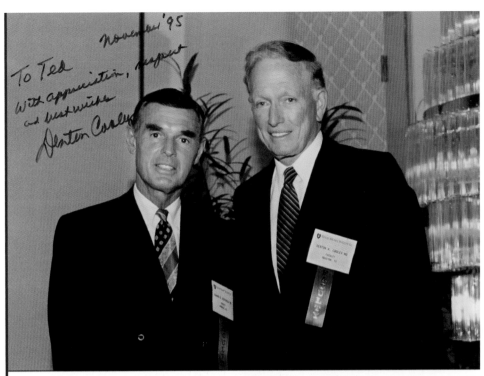

Dr. Cooley and me at an International Congress meeting in Phoenix in 1995 when he was presented the Lifetime Achievement Award by the Arizona Heart Foundation.

This supplement was distributed to all of the attendees, and a standing ovation honored this great pioneer.

Dr. Volodos was not credited with performing the first endovascular repair of an abdominal aortic aneurysm because it was not recorded in the English literature. Therefore, the credit goes to Dr. Juan Parodi from Buenos Aires for his procedure in 1991. Juan and I became friends and later exchanged many ideas relative to this new technology. In fact, I developed endografts in our laboratories, which later became commercial products.

Stop the presses. 2015. Endologix has just announced a merger with TriVascular, another giant in the endoluminal graft sector. Read on in Chapter 40 of an elderly woman in Colorado with a ruptured abdominal aneurysm, critical and near death. She was flown to the Arizona Heart Hospital where the homemade endograft was being sterilized for deployment in a life-saving effort. The next day

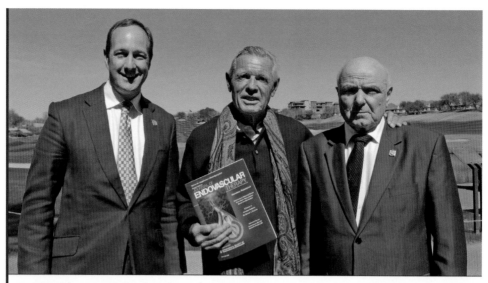

In 2013, the International Society of Endovascular Specialists honored Professor Nikolay L. Volodos—shown here with me, and Mr. Reid, the President of the Society. It is quite clear who lives in Arizona and who in the northern environs of Scotland and the Ukraine.

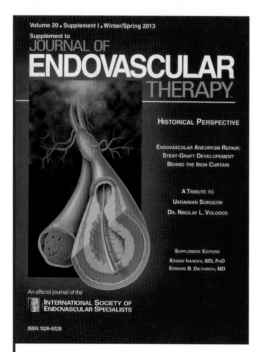

Volume 20 • Supplement I • Winter/Spring 2013

Supplement to

JOURNAL OF
ENDOVASCULAR
THERAPY.

HISTORICAL PERSPECTIVE

ENDOVASCULAR ANEURYSM REPAIR:
STENT-GRAFT DEVELOPEMENT
BEHIND THE IRON CURTAIN

A TRIBUTE TO
UKRAINIAN SURGEON
DR. NIKOLAY L. VOLODOS

SUPPLEMENT EDITORS
KRASSI IVANCEV, MD, PhD
EDWARD B. DIETHRICH, MD

An official journal of the
**INTERNATIONAL SOCIETY OF
ENDOVASCULAR SPECIALISTS**

ISSN 1526-6028

A special supplement of the journal was published detailing Professor Volodos' early accomplishments in the field of endovascular surgery.

the patient told the story, "Oh I don't have the pain…" This amalgamation is further testimony to my consistent search of therapies, techniques, and opportunities to deliver treatment of heart and blood vessel disease.

At our International Congress VII in 1994, I decided to do a live case demonstration of an endovascular procedure. To my knowledge, it had not been performed live. While I was considering the selection of an appropriate patient, my good friend Dino Tatooles from Chicago called to obtain my opinion on one of his patients. He had heard me lecture on

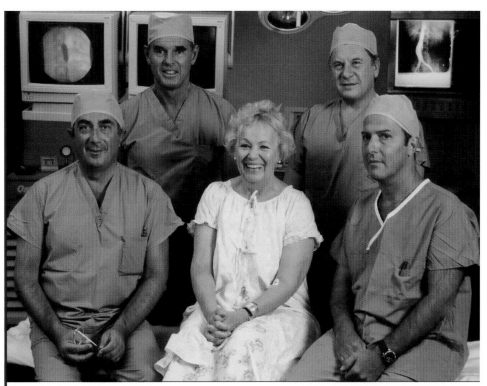

The first live EVAR (endovascular aneurysm repair) case during the International Congress VII in 1994. The patient, Lorraine Mascari, is flanked by Dr. Juan Parodi (left) and Dr. Claudio Schönholz (right). I am in the back beside Dr. Tatooles who brought the patient to Phoenix from Chicago.

the subject, and he mailed me the patient films. She seemed like a good candidate for endovascular surgery, and Dino felt her heart condition placed her at high risk for the open procedure. In the end, she came to Phoenix, and we performed the procedure live for an auditorium packed with physicians from around the world. I invited Juan and our friend Claudio Schönholz to participate in this historic event.

Two years after our first live demonstration for treatment of an abdominal aortic aneurysm with an endograft, Michael Dake MD, an interventional radiologist, at that time working at Stanford University, described the first use of endografts for aneurysmal disease in the thoracic aorta.

Dr. Dake today is Professor of Cardiovascular Surgery at Stanford, which is testimony that the specialty amalgamation has truly occurred.

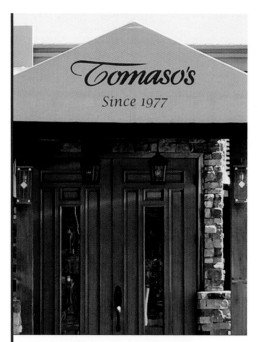

Site of another serendipitous event.

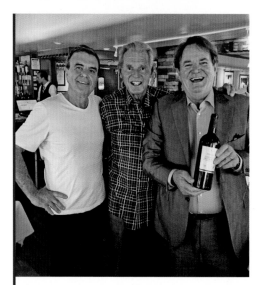

Tommy Tomaso (left) and I are revisiting my first introduction to Tony Niccoli. He was also chatting with Armando De Zan, CEO and Owner of AREL GROUP, Wine & Spirits, Inc. At the conclusion of the lunch, Tommy said, "Doc, you do recommend red wine for the heart don't you?"

I traveled to California to observe Mike's work and participated in the Gore protocol, which Mike spearheaded. In that regard, we ended up with a common patient. I was eating dinner at one of my favorite restaurants in Phoenix, of course, an Italian one, when the owner, Tommy came up to talk to me.

"Doctor, I want you to meet a gentleman in the next room."

He ushered me to another table and introduced me to Tony Niccoli, a local businessman. We had an interesting conversation that ended with a completely unexpected result. Tony was interested in hearing about my work, particularly that relating to research and new technology. I explained to him the current status of our ultrasound company, ADR. He was intrigued in the business aspects and inquired about my expectations for the company in the future. He immediately suggested that ADR was a very marketable company for one of the larger instrument corporations looking for new products. We met on several occasions later but the end result was the sale of the company orchestrated by Tony.

Tony and I developed a great friendship and when he mentioned on one occasion that he had been diagnosed with a thoracic aneurysm and had heard of Dr. Dake's work, I suggested he set up an appointment for treatment with the new thoracic endograft.

That actually occurred, and I informed Mike that we would perform follow-up studies here in Phoenix.

Today, this is one of the most successful techniques we have to treat disease of the thoracic aorta. It became more popular with the introduction

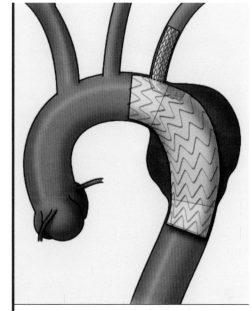

The Gore thoracic endograft used to accomodate flow through the left subclavian branch.

of vascular closure devices (VCDs). These devices are used to seal the artery in the groin where the endograft is inserted, replacing the need for an incision and open exposure of the artery.

Zvonimir Krajcer, MD, Clinical Professor at Baylor College of Medicine, is one of the leaders in this VCD technology. We have worked together in various capacities over the years and are very close friends. He is the President-elect for the International Society of Endovascular Specialists. I am confident he will do an outstanding job in that new position.

The evolution of endovascular therapy created a molding of the scientific clinician and the corporate partner in the world of new devices. The board of ISES was the perfect example of that amalgamation with the industry partners joining the various medical specialties. Marv Woodall was a corporate executive who understood and fully appreciated the clinical practice.

Zvonko Krajcer, MD.

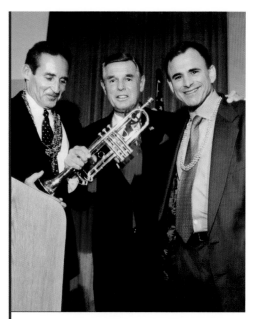

Trumpet presented to me at the NCVH conference in 2002.

The Palmaz stent became an integral component of our endovascular armamentarium. Julio Palmaz was an interventional radiologist in San Antonio, Texas. Richard Schatz, MD, after leaving the military, joined Julio and this led to the Palmaz-Schatz coronary stent.

Dr. Schatz joined us in Phoenix and directed our efforts for both peripheral and coronary stent opportunities in the FDA clinical trials. In fact, AHI had the largest single center enrollment in the iliac stent approval process. Clearly, this was a major differentiator for the program. Richard ultimately went to Scripps Clinic in San Diego, where he has had a very successful career. It is certain that the Palmaz-Schatz stent would not have been released in 1994 without Marv's personal efforts and dedication in spearheading the stent technology.

I have been most fortunate to know and work with Marv these many years. As a leader of the ISES board, he most recently took the lead role in acquiring our

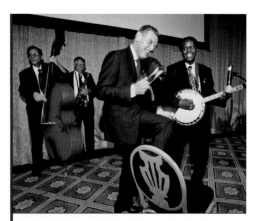

Demonstrating my spoon playing to the NCVH attendees.

new publisher, SAGE, for the *Journal of Endovascular Therapy*. He continues to be a leading force today at the board level.

However, not all of my colleagues on the ISES board and its members in general were in agreement that the endovascular society would indeed need to be multidisciplinary, with surgeons, cardiologists, radiologists, and more. But the movement was on, and other major conferences and meetings on the topic were springing up. One of the most important and distinguished meetings, is the New Cardiovascular Horizons (NCVH) conference held in New Orleans as well as the multiple regional meetings that organization holds throughout the year. The genius behind this effort is Dr. Craig Walker from Houma, Louisiana. I had the great pleasure to

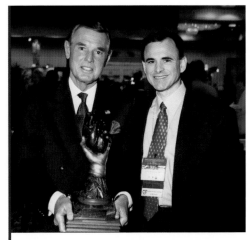

Custom bronze award from my good friend, Craig Walker.

be honored at this meeting in New Orleans in 2002. Interestingly, he presented a trumpet but did not ask me to perform.

He and his group were more interested in my ability to play the spoons. (Yes, during medical school and my internship I had a spoon band that played to counter the stress of our work.)

In addition, Craig presented me with a beautiful bronze sculpture of the human heart.

ISES continues to have a close relationship with Dr. Walker and his team as he remains a driving force in the cardiovascular arena. His philosophy reflects that of ISES, where close cooperation between industrial partners and academia is a huge component in fostering rapid growth of new concepts and bringing them to fruition.

38

September 11ᵗʰ The Great Escape, Route 66

The phone rang precisely at 7 a.m., just as I had instructed the hotel operator the night before. I said thanks before my usual spring out of bed. I went to the window to check the weather. It was a clear blue sky in Washington, DC, where I was to deliver some papers at the Annual TCT (Transcatheter Cardiovascular Therapeutics) meeting in the Washington Convention Center next to the Hyatt. Several thousand registrants were anticipated for the international meeting.

After the usual toiletries I went to the first floor where a speaker-ready room was set up for presenters to review their slides and make last minute changes. There were about ten to fifteen colleagues already at the computer stations when I arrived. I was sipping a coffee waiting in line when my phone rang.

"Are you watching TV?" The question rang in my ear from my office in Phoenix. I did not even have time to reply, "Turn it on! At 8:46 a.m. American Airlines Flight 11 left from Boston for Los Angeles and crashed into the North Tower of the World Trade Center, killing everyone on board and several hundred inside the building!"

I clicked off the connection and immediately turned on the large television in the prep room. I could not believe my eyes. Almost spontaneously I turned to the gang assembled at their computers. "A plane crashed into the World Trade Center!" I shouted.

The computer screens went blank. Every ear in the room suddenly was attached to a cell phone and all eyes focused on the large screen in the room. No wonder it was almost impossible to make phone calls anywhere just ten minutes later. I quickly ran to the front door and out on the street toward the convention hall. It was a mass exodus. Everyone was shouting, "No meeting, the Trade Center is under lockdown!" I turned around and raced to the prep room, but it was already completely empty. Just slide trays next to blank computer screens. I continued to watch television as it was announced that United Airlines Flight 175, which left Boston bound for Los Angeles, crashed into the WTC's South Tower at 9:03 a.m. I suddenly felt very alone. How could this be happening to my America?

I went to the hotel lobby where many of my friends were mingling around large TV sets. Dr. Rodney White and Paul McCormick from Endologix sat down next to me with a Starbucks coffee. At 9:31 a.m. President Bush announced that the events in New York City were apparent terrorist attacks on our country. At 9:37 a.m., American Airlines Flight 77 from Dulles bound for Los Angeles crashed into The Pentagon in Washington, DC, killing 59 aboard and 125 military and civilian personnel in the building. The entire city was being affected.

Our conversation was frequented with frustration, apprehension, and sadness. After a couple of hours and many more heartbreaking shots on television, we decided to locate a place for lunch, even though I don't believe any of us had much of an appetite. At 9:59 a.m. the news reported that the South Tower of the WTC collapsed. Sirens were screeching outside the hotel. Then the TV showed more bad news: the WTC's North Tower collapsed at 10:28 a.m.

Our lunch turned out to be a planning session because the city was certainly heading toward lockdown. The first item on our impromptu agenda was how to get out of Washington as quickly as possible.

At 9 a.m. at his home near Philadelphia, Bob Fultano's son told him there was a plane accident in NYC. Bob thought it was a small plane and paid little attention. However, at 9:30 a.m., Bob received the crucial call from Paul McCormick, his boss who had joined us in the lobby. It was the first that Bob had heard of the disastrous news of NYC and Washington, DC.

We decided to split the duties in order to execute the plan "How to Escape Washington." At this point we had four on the team: Dr. Rodney White from UCLA, Paul McCormick from Endologix, me, and a scientist who had just sat down at our table. Not wanting to insult him, I asked him to join the team. Rod would check on trains and buses. I would explore the potential for rental cars. Paul was assigned to check on airline availabilities. Dr. Tom Fogarty, world famous inventor and cardiovascular surgeon, suddenly sat down; however, his association with the group was brief. After the planning session, he was nowhere to be found. We agreed to meet at 4 p.m. to compare results of our assignments, which turned out to be a series of zeros. No planes, no trains, no buses, and no rental cars. There were still vacant hotel rooms, but those were filling rapidly. All members provided good but rather desperate reports.

Paul showed the ingenuity of his corporate position. Bob Fultano, now fully aware of the situation, was key to our escape. He went directly to an Enterprise car rental agency, rented an SUV, and proceeded on Highway 95S to DC, which was usually a trip of two to two-and-a-half hours. That morning it was a much quicker drive; there was absolutely no traffic at all. However, all bridges and the Baltimore tunnel were flocked with military Humvees. Upon arrival in DC, Bob saw even more of a military presence, including Humvees with machine guns and light tanks, along with helicopters and F-16 type jets in the sky. He said it was a very eerie feeling.

Bob parked on a side street next to the Hyatt. We loaded quickly, and then expressed our independent opinions on where to go. The final consensus was that we should head west, "yes go west, young men, go west."

We revved the engine and the trip was on. Soon we were passing the residence of the Vice President of the United States at the Naval Observatory. I'm sure he was not at home; most likely in a deep bunker somewhere off site, certainly far from where President Bush was in isolation.

Our first destination was Cleveland, Ohio. Our plan was to drop the car off and grab the next plane to the West Coast. Little did we know that at 9:42 a.m. that morning, for the first time in the history of the FAA, all flights in the United

States and Canada were grounded, totaling about 3,300 commercial and 1,200 private aircraft. There were no airplanes in the sky, except military or those cleared by President Bush. Several hours later we pulled up at a hotel near the Cleveland airport and received word that Cleveland airport was closed.

We decided to head southwest toward St. Louis and drove straight on the I-70, thinking the farther from Washington and NYC the better. By the time we reached St. Louis, the hunger pangs had begun. I chose the restaurant, an Italian one, and ordered a fine bottle of Ruffino. Bob refused a sip because he was to be the next driver in the rotation.

Rod was sitting next to me at the table. As the discussion continued, we realized there was a strong possibility that we might not find a flight for some time. Rod and I looked at each other. Neither one of us were too interested in staying for who knows how long in a surrounding motel. The others did not seem to care so much. The executive decision was made to drive to the West Coast non-stop, except for gas and bathroom breaks. And that is exactly what we did.

By this time we had set up rotations for driving in only two to three hour shifts. We passed through Missouri without incident, but in eastern Oklahoma, where traffic slowed, there was some kind of checkpoint in response to 9/11. Here we were, the four of us, in a car rented two days before in a city 1,400 miles away. What made it worse was that Bob was bald, wearing black glasses and a two-day beard growth. He looked mighty suspicious.

We put him on the floor behind the front seat and covered the disguised agent with our coats. We made it through. I guess we didn't look like terrorists, but the driving rotations were changed. Rod and I thought Paul drove too slowly. Bob thought my speeds of 105 mph were excessive. Nevertheless, Rod and I took over. Paul could sleep the rest of the way to Flagstaff.

No one in our quartet was a great navigator, and furthermore none of us had ever driven from the East Coast to the West Coast. It seemed obvious, however, that from St. Louis we knew to go southwest and directly on to Arizona. It turned out to be the course of the original Historic Route 66.

In 2014, while in New York City for the Veith meeting, I passed one of those stands that sells everything from hot dogs to snow caps. At first I missed it, but on a turnaround, there was the historic sign of Route 66. I quickly snapped a photo on my cell phone to remind me of our own historic trip.

Had we known of Route 66 and the famous song about it, we no doubt would have been singing all the way to Flagstaff:

"If you ever plan to motor west,

Travel my way, take the highway that is best.

Get your kicks on route sixty-six.

It winds from Chicago to LA,

More than two thousand miles all the way.

Get your kicks on route sixty-six.

Now you go through Saint Looey

Joplin, Missouri,

And Oklahoma City is mighty pretty.

Even without a plan, we ended up on Historic Route 66 leading to Arizona.

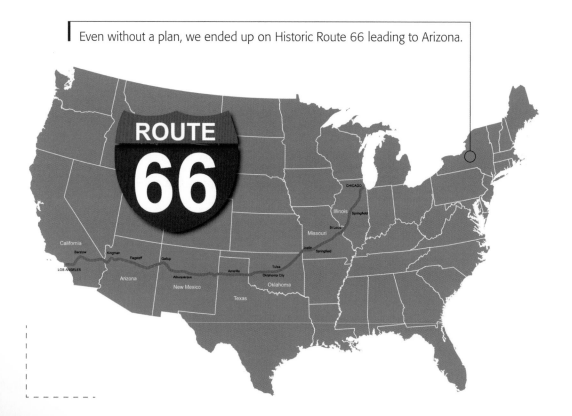

You see Amarillo,

Gallup, New Mexico,

Flagstaff, Arizona.

Don't forget Winona,

Kingman, Barstow, San Bernardino.

Won't you get hip to this timely tip:

When you make that California trip

Get your kicks on route sixty-six.

Won't you get hip to this timely tip:

When you make that California trip

Get your kicks on route sixty-six.

Get your kicks on route sixty-six.

Get your kicks on route sixty-six."

As the trip progressed our cell phone batteries became nearly depleted, but I did get one message through to my secretary in Phoenix and made arrangements for her to meet me in Flagstaff. The others went on to LAX and beyond after dropping me off.

That was the story of our great escape of 9/11. It was a day of shock and anger with sadness, and a time of terror. In the end, though, the nation came back stronger and wiser, despite the unimaginable death toll. The bravery of many was exhibited as well.

As Bush expressed when he addressed the nation: "These acts of mass murder were intended to frighten our nation into chaos and retreat. But they have failed. Our country is strong. A great people have been moved to defend a great nation. Terrorist attacks can shake the foundations of our biggest buildings, but they cannot touch the foundation of America. These acts shatter steel, but they cannot dent the steel of American resolve."

Today, some fourteen years later, I am not at all convinced our leadership understands the message of 9/11. 911 denotes an emergency!

39

Mamma Mia—A Dream Come

When I wrote Chapter 15 on "Heart" Felt Dreams it resonates my conversation with Tommy Thompson, the author of *Hearts*. It had a side note relating to Dr. Cooley and his aspirations and reflects the obvious differences between generations.

It is now apparent that those dreams were in the embryonic stage of maturation. They also did not anticipate what I would face in Phoenix with the medical community and later on with much of the establishment of vascular surgery. I was young and I was a dreamer but without absolute realization of what it would take to succeed in my life. I am sure that my colleagues in medicine, as well as other professions, have experienced similar circumstances.

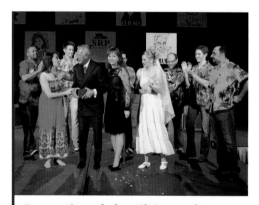

Presentation of the Lifetime Achievement Award (Phoenix Theatre) to me by Linda Pope, Arizona Heart Foundation Board member (right) along with the cast of *Mamma Mia*.

In 2013, an event occurred that amalgamated whatever scattered thinking I might have been experiencing.

The Phoenix Theater came to visit me with the news that I had been selected for the annual Lifetime Achievement Award. This was unusual because I had never been active with the theater. However, they obviously

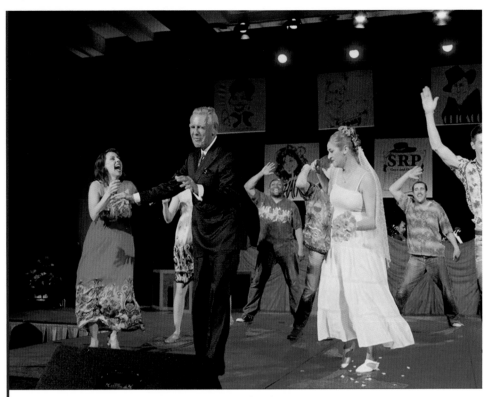

I am singing a song from *Mamma Mia* with the theatre group.

knew of my love for music, and during the interview they asked about my favorite musical. My instant response was *Mamma Mia.* They did not inquire why nor did I explain. On the evening of the affair, my family and friends were seated directly below the round stage.

As the presentation ensued, the music began and singers and actors took the stage, singing the music of ABBA *Mamma Mia.* As the conclusion drew near, the singers formed a semi-circle directly above our table, and with full chorus sang the final song "I Have a Dream" right above my head:

> I have a dream, a song to sing
> To help me cope with anything
> If you see the wonder of a fairy tale
> You can take the future, even if you fail

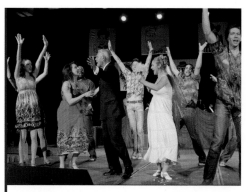

Dancing with the performers after receiving the award.

I believe in angels, something good in everything I see
I believe in angels, when I know the time is right for me
I'll cross the stream
I have a dream

I have a dream, a fantasy
To help me through reality
And my destination makes it worth the while
Pushing through the darkness, still another mile

I believe in angels, something good in everything I see
I believe in angels when I know the time is right for me
I'll cross the stream
I have a dream

They escorted me onto the stage, where the musicians were still singing. I took the liberty to do a few dance steps with the actors.

Could there have been anything more appropriate to capsulize my life in receiving this lifetime achievement award?

At the right time, I did cross the stream and fulfill my dream.

40

Power of Three—
To Care, To Teach, To Pioneer

On the wall of our classroom at the Arizona Heart Institute where the entire staff met each Thursday morning, three words were inscribed on the wall: "To Care, To Teach, To Pioneer." It was certainly a laudable mission for guiding a young surgeon's journey to the future. The details of the road map were sometimes a bit blurred, but the ultimate goal was always crystal clear: to mold three specific missions into a structure that would provide the maximum opportunity for success for the goals of each. We recognized the physical components that were critical to the organization of the triad—we called it the "Power of Three."

Arizona Heart Institute—An outpatient cardiovascular center where, underneath one roof, the most contemporary diagnostic equipment and delivery of patient care was provided. It was truly a unique entity, giving physicians the ability to review tests and provide a plan of action for their patients the same day. This exemplified the Ist Power.

The Arizona Heart Hospital—An adjacent specialty facility with patient

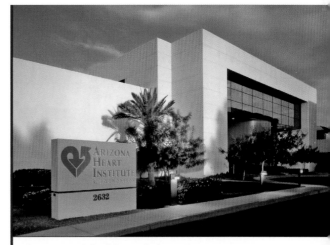

The second building of the Arizona Heart Institute, one block south of the Arizona Heart Hospital.

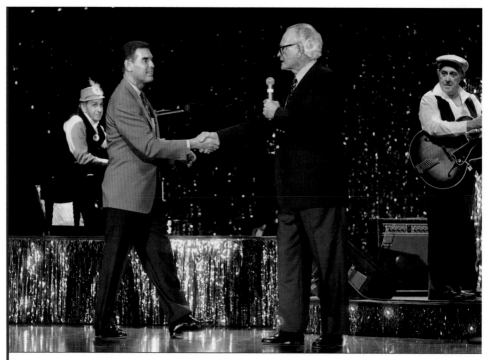

Barry Goldwater with me in the auditorium at the Sun Dome Stadium in Sun City where 5,000 attended a special presentation by the Arizona Heart Institute called the "Celebration of the Heart." I performed coronary surgery on the senator the year before. He became a friend and was a strong supporter of the AHI programs.

care focusing exclusively on the treatment of heart and blood vessel disease. A true specialty hospital, only the second in the United States, that exemplified a Center of Excellence with incomparable patient care. This represented the 2nd Power.

The transitional administrative team that made this move successful was Karen DeWitt, President of the hospital; Sue Carroll, RN, Vice President of Clinical Services; and Chris Winters, Vice President of Finance.

And finally…

The Translational Research Center—The investigative initiative in the "Power of Three" afforded a unique opportunity to take an embryonic idea and nurture it all the way to clinical application. A true bench-to-bedside experience. This epitome of translational research represented the 3rd Power. These three elements completed the campus, and permitted execution of our mission: To Care, To Teach, and To Pioneer.

This "Power of Three" structure was highly successful in providing diagnosis and treatment for patients who came to us from around the world. The techniques and procedures being developed were shared with both young and established physicians in the cardiovascular arena. Clearly, the annual cardiovascular congresses, most recently known as iCON, drew from near and far and were duplicated in other continents as far away as China. The China project was aggressive in nature since it was proposed to essentially duplicate the Arizona Heart Institute model in Beijing. It would have been a great tribute to the Institute vision; however,

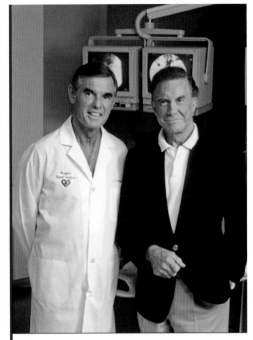

The famous actor, Cliff Robertson, was one of the Arizona Heart Foundation's most active members. He narrated several movies and often spoke at educational meetings. He was also a close personal friend of my family and me.

the partnership between Phoenix and Beijing could not be brought to fruition. A successful project was Vivo Petrov's conference in Sophia, Bulgaria, where I inaugurated the City Clinic with the Prime Minister.

Today, as I visit programs around the world, it is rewarding to meet the many trainees that we had the unique opportunity to educate and share our visions for the future. The positive movement of the endovascular approach to treating disease that we espoused early on is now revered as exemplified by the suc-

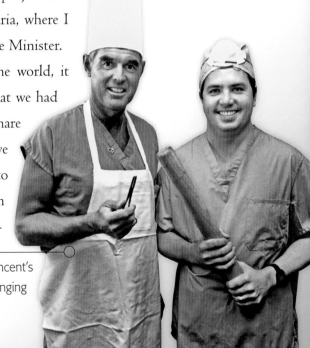

Two masters—board member and owner of Vincent's Restaurant, Vincent Guerithault, and me exchanging our secrets.

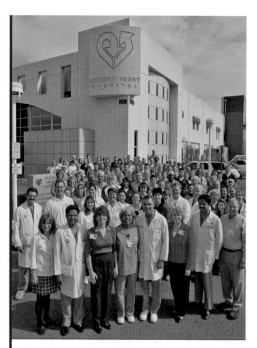

The Arizona Heart Hospital, established in 1998, is dedicated exclusively to cardiovascular treatment in the United States. Here, the entire staff is proudly celebrating its grand opening.

cess of the International Society of Endovascular Specialists and its publication, the Journal of Endovascular Therapy. However, a physical plant is irrelevant if void of people dedicated to the campus mission. In that regard I was most fortunate.

From the beginning to the end of my active surgical career, I was blessed to have some of the most wonderfully dedicated staff, willing to face every barrier with a solution and every success with a celebration. These individuals contributed greatly to our program.

Greg Petras was the financial engineer who directed the dollars

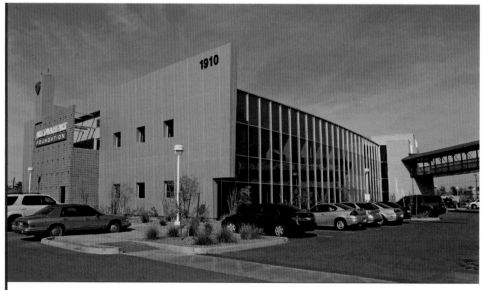

The Arizona Heart Foundation, home of the School of Cardiac & Vascular Ultrasound, built in 2006.

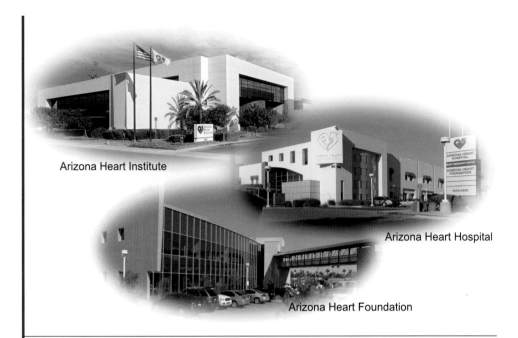

Arizona Heart Institute

Arizona Heart Hospital

Arizona Heart Foundation

The Power of Three: The Arizona Heart Institute, The Arizona Heart Hospital, and The Translational Research and Education Center, now the home of the Arizona Heart Foundation. The influence of the Power of Three was quick to expand beyond the borders of Arizona to international sites.

and cents of the operation. He went on to create his own company, which was wildly successful.

Dewey Schade was retiring from the military when he sent me a letter describing his enthusiasm for my vision, which he had witnessed in *Hearts*. He became a loyal employee and established the International Advisory Board of the Institute. This board was made up of some of the most important business people in the world, for example: Robert Marston, of Marston & Assoc. in NYC who was very helpful in our marketing strategies and public relations. Its value in our early years cannot be overestimated.

At the time of my interview with the ethics committee of the Maricopa Medical Society upon entering Phoenix, I did not have, either in mind or on paper, a specific public relations or marketing plan for the Arizona Heart Institute. I was already committed to a strong audiovisual department, VAS, but much ground

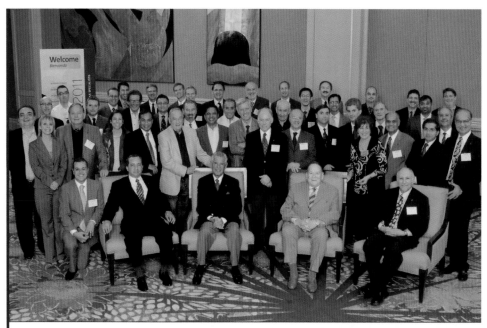

The Edward B. Diethrich Vascular Surgical Society 2011 meeting, seated from left to right: Leonardo Lucas, Marwan Ghazoul, Edward B. Diethrich, Roger Greenhalgh, Alfonso Munoz. First row standing left to right: Armando Lobato, Dawn Olsen, Claudio Zamorano, Nadia Vallejo, Venkatesh Ramaiah, Thomas Fogarty, Rajagopalan Ravi, Jacques Bleyn, Jay Kiessling, Giancarlo Accarino, Henry Tarlian, Erika Scott, Ravi Koopot, Dilip Bobra, Hara Misra. Second row standing: Mark Rummel, Alexandro Mallios, Konstantinos Konstantinidis, Patrick Peeters, Khaja Moinuddeen, Rodney White, Ali AbuRahma, Lucien Castellani, Ying Wei Lum, Surya Kumar, Alan Werner, Edmond Raker, Chandrahas Patel, Luis Lopez-Galarza. Last row: Alexander Bueno Silva, Kelston DeSales, Julio Rodriguez, Matthew Namanny, James May, Jacques Busquet, Alberto Benassi, Donald Reid, Dwain Stone, David Caparrelli, Christopher Kwolek, Stephen Greenhalgh. I cherish the photograph and the smiling faces of so many of my colleagues and fellows I have trained around the world.

work had to be plotted, certainly a state component to our International Advisory Board would be critical to our ultimate plan. As in any organization, the individual contributors are key to success.

Locally, where I had not even begun to approach the war to come, key positive communication was vital. Pat McMahon was a famous local radio and TV host. He became the third man on the Wallace & Ladmo program that had aired nearly 10,000 episodes before ending in 1989. He was a natural at the microphone and became a devoted spokesperson for the AHF program. Most important, Pat believed in our mission and fully understood that public education was critical to the fight against cardiovascular disease. I appeared frequently on his shows, and when we introduced the Mr. Heart program to the schools, Pat was a strong supporter. I have never received a negative response from Pat to any of my multiple requests for his assistance over all these years.

Lance Lewis, a son of a former judge in Pennsylvania, joined us to

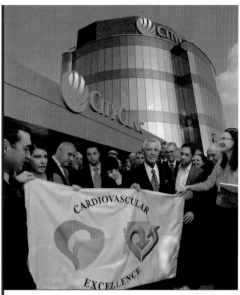

The City Clinic. I am holding the banner with our combined logos on it for the new City Clinic.

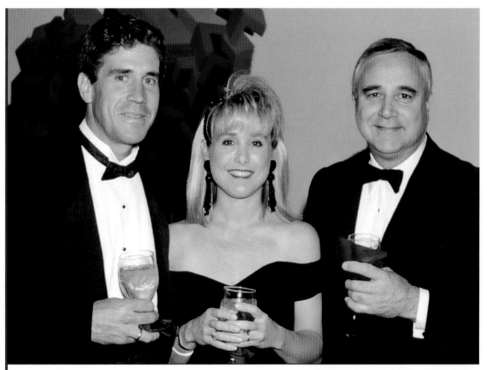

Robert Marston, far right, a key member of the Institute's National Advisory Board, celebrating at a special event of the Foundation with my daughter Lynne and her husband Joe Jackson.

organize the AHI State Advisory Board. When the Great War was upon us, this board provided the fodder to fight off the enemy.

I will be forever indebted to these three monumental contributors to our success. Three different people who represented different disciplines, all united to contribute to the Power of Three. They truly reflected our mission: To Care, To Teach, To Pioneer.

There are innumerable examples extolling the virtues of the Power of Three concept. Because of my interest in biomedical engineering, our work tended to lean toward the newer technologies for treating aneurysmal disease in a less invasive manner. Joining us to concentrate almost exclusively in this research was cardiovascular surgeon Dr. Myles Douglas. Our effort became a true example of bench-to-bedside. Using his device, concept models were built and tested on the bench to perfect both the delivery of the device and also its ability to exclude the aneurysm from the circulation.

Our next step was to apply it to the animal models using the same testing principles but also examining long-term survival in order to have histological data on the materials and their interface with the arterial wall. These were the same studies being performed by others worldwide as the endovascular concept gained momentum. I have always been very proud of the fellows who came from outside the US to train with our program; Dr. Papazoglou from Greece (referred to in the AHI Abroad and Athens chapters) was

Pat McMahon showing off with Mr. Heart.

a classic example. From the southern hemisphere came three Chilean doctors: Luis A. Munoz, Claudio Zamorano, and Louis Coppelli. They moved to Payson, Arizona, after their fellowship year to establish a surgical practice. Dr. Munoz later became President of the Edward B. Diethrich Vascular Surgical Society. He exhibited great leadership skills to parallel his operative acumen.

Claudio Zamorano and I also had

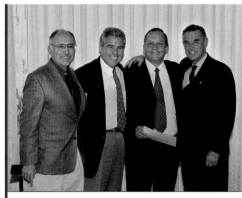

My three Chilean Vascular Fellows formed a new society in my honor. From left to right are Dr. Munoz, Dr. Coppelli, Dr. Zamorano, and me.

a personal relationship in that we both played the trumpet. Claudio even started a jazz band in Payson and frequently they would play for occasions at the Institute. Several years ago, he decided to return to Chile and I presented him with my Al Hirt trumpet. I was certain he would do great musical credit south of the border. Just last week he stopped in to see me on a visit to his friends in Payson. He has formed another jazz band in Santiago and the notes from Al's trumpet are the highlight of the group. Once again medicine and music are joined.

One morning I received an urgent phone call from a physician in Cortez, Colorado, who had an elderly lady with a ruptured aneurysm. He felt she would

not last long, but was not comfortable with operating due to the complexity of the case and her general health. We made arrangements for an air ambulance transfer to the Heart Hospital. This was truly an emergency situation to save a life.

Immediately I had the nurse page Myles, as he was in the laboratory. "Myles, there is a ruptured abdominal

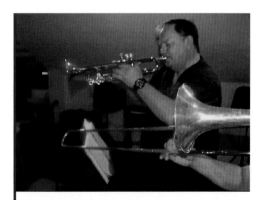

The jazz band performing at Club de Jazz de Santiago, featuring Claudio Zamorano playing the Al Hirt trumpet.

aneurysm being flown in. She is in desperate shape and an extremely poor risk for an open operation. I believe we should treat her with the new endograft," I explained. It did not take any convincing; he was probably getting tired of all the pre-clinical experimentation. I headed to the operating room and explained our plans.

Next I called VAS. This was going to be a first, and I wanted it documented for posterity. We met the helicopter on the pad at the emergency door and headed directly to the operating room. Cameras were covering the entire event, including documentation of all the time intervals between the various stages. The procedure was executed perfectly, just as we had rehearsed so many times before. There was no blood loss, there were no transfusions. The next morning on rounds I asked the patient how she was feeling.

"Oh I feel fine. That terrible pain is all gone."

It was a success! We did complete the surgical movie, and later used it for educational purposes.

A couple of days later I called Mike Henson in California. He had been president of the hot tip laser company, Trimedyne, when I was working on that project. I told him I had a must-see operative case. He flew in the next morning. Myles and I showed him our experimental work and answered his questions before I rolled the film of the operation. Serendipity in action.

Together we formed a new company named Endologix. This company still exists and has many products in the field of cardiovascular medicine. This company is an example of how proud I am of the people who have worked with me over the years. It's not only the physicians who have passed through our program who gave me a feeling of success, but also the nurses, technicians, paramedical personnel, and even the members of industry who have melded into our society of endovascular specialists. One who particularly stands out is Robert Wrasper, who was a radiology technician during the early days of intra-operative arteriography. Today he stands high on the list of clinical specialists in the Endologix Corporation.

Would we dare repeat that experiment today? Of course not! Does that negative response suggest it was an incorrect thing to do? I sincerely doubt it. The basic tenet of serendipity is freedom to explore, unencumbered by external restrictions and constraints. But that's a subject for another book.

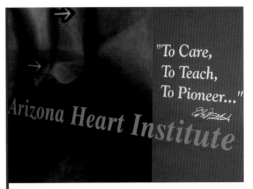

"To Care, To Teach, To Pioneer"—the mission of the AHF.

The corporate hospital partner with whom we were so successful in building the Power of Three made the decision to sell its interests to another health care company. A total management and culture change occurred overnight. The first morning after the corporate exchange, the new management called a meeting of all the employees, physicians included. We were crowded into the third floor classroom, where "To Care, To Teach, To Pioneer" was inscribed on the wall.

I was seated, quietly discussing work with some of the other doctors, when the leader of the meeting introduced herself and proceeded to tell the staff "how things were going to be different from this point on." I never anticipated how different it would eventually become until she said, "From this day forward there will be no free services to any patient. All patients not covered by insurance would either make arrangements to pay personally or the service would not be provided." I stood up. It was impossible for me to contain myself.

"Miss Somebody, (I don't remember her name because I immediately erased it from my memory bank forever. She is not even in my contact list.) that will not be acceptable to the doctors. I have practiced in this city since 1971 and have never, ever refused to treat a patient because of financial circumstances. In fact, at my early morning clinic (the EBD Clinic referenced earlier), I have never submitted a professional fee for the consultations; only for those where I had performed a procedure was a bill sent or insurance form submitted." My words fell on deaf ears.

She replied, "Doctor, this is your new environment and we set the rules." Indeed, we were like strangers groping in the dark. The core of the AHI mission had been destroyed in the single stroke of a pen…my pen when I signed the contract.

I am quoting Hippocrates "The Physician's Oath" at this point to show the dramatic contrast between what we as physicians pledged and what the new ownership demanded.

"The Physician's Oath"

Some followers of Hippocrates of Cos (fl.430 BC) may have taken this sacred oath, which regulated the conduct of the healer as well as his "professional" obligations. Works of surgery do appear in the large Hippocratic corpus, amassed between 400 and 100 BC, and thus many of the Coan School were not bound to this code. Hippocrates himself surely did not write the oath:

I swear by Apollo Physician and Asclepius and Hygieia and Panaceia and all the gods and goddesses, making them my witnesses, that I will fulfill according to my ability and judgment this oath and this covenant:

To hold him who has taught me this art as equal to my parents and to live my life in partnership with him, and if he is in need of money to give him a share of mine, and to regard his offspring as equal to my brothers in male lineage and to teach them this art—if they desire to learn it—without fee and covenant; to give a share of precepts and oral instruction and all other learning to my sons and to the sons of him who has instructed me and to pupils who have signed the covenant and have taken an oath according to the medical law, but to no one else.

I will apply dietetic measures for the benefit of the sick according to my ability and judgment; I will keep them from harm and injustice.

I will neither give a deadly drug to anybody if asked for it, nor will I make a suggestion to this effect. Similarly I will not give to a woman an abortive remedy. In purity and holiness I will guard my life and my art.

I will not use the knife, not even on sufferers from stone, but will withdraw in favor of such men as are engaged in this work.

Whatever houses I may visit, I will come for the benefit of the sick, remaining free of all intentional injustice, of all mischief and in particular of sexual relations with both female and male persons, be they free or slaves.

What I may see or hear in the course of treatment or even outside of the treatment in regard to the life of men, which on no account one must spread abroad, I will keep to myself holding such things shameful to be spoken about.

If I fulfill this oath and do not violate it, many it be granted to me to enjoy life and art, being honored with fame among all men for all time to come; if I transgress it and swear falsely, may the opposite of all this be my lot.

In light of the new corporate policy I found it to be more appropriate to expose a modern version of the oath, probably to be more consistent with the philosophy of our new bosses.

This parodist selection originally appeared in a publication called *The Journal of Irreproducible Results* by? Anonymous, MD.

Revised Hippocratic Oath—

I swear by Apollo the physician, by Aesculapius, by Melvin Belli, and by my DEA number, to keep according to the advice of my accountant and attorney the following oath:

To consider dear to me as my stock certificates him who enabled me to learn this art: the banker who approved my educational loans; to live in common with him and to acquire my mortgages through his bank and that of his sons; to consider equally dear my teachers, and if necessary to split fees with them and request from them unnecessary consultations. I will prescribe regimen for the good of my practice according to my patients' third party coverage or remaining Medicaid stickers, taking care not to perform non-reimbursable procedures. To please no one, with the possible exception of favored detail men, will I prescribe a non-FDA approved drug unless it should be essential to one of my clinical research projects; nor will I give advice which may cause my patient's death prior to obtaining a flat EEG for 24 hours. But I will preserve the purity of my reputation. In every clinical situation, I will cover my ass by ordering all conceivable lab work and by documenting my every move in the chart. I will faithfully accumulate 25 Category I CME credits per year, and none of these by attending Sports Medicine conferences on the slopes of Aspen. I will not cut for stone, even for patients in whom the disease is manifest, before documenting the diagnosis by I.V. or retrograde pyelogram and obtaining informed consent. In every house where I come I will enter only if a house call is absolutely unavoidable, keeping myself far from all intentional ill-doing and all seduction, and especially free from the pleasures of love with women or with men. Or, for that matter, with both simultaneously. Such activities I will confine to my office or yacht. I will not be induced to testify against my colleagues in court, nor to disagree with them when asked for a second opinion. I will not charge less for any procedure than the prevailing rate in my community. All that may come to my knowledge in the exercise of my profession, such as diagnoses, prognoses, detail of treatment and fee schedules, I will keep secret and never reveal to patients; I will, however, cheerfully provide these to insurance companies. Finally, under no circumstances will I vote for Ted Kennedy or anyone else of his ilk. If I keep this oath faithfully, may I enjoy my life, build my practice, incorporate, find some solid tax shelters, and ultimately make a killing in real estate; but if I swerve from it or violate it, may a profusion of malpractice claims be my lot.

This new environment was completely foreign to us and inconsistent with the oath we had taken in becoming doctors. Yes, I have to take the blame. But in my defense, the original acquiring company had their agent in my office several times a week, saying, "Don't worry, doctor, there will be no significant changes in the program. Everything will operate as usual after the transaction."

I should have listened to the reporter from the *Business Journal* when I conveyed to her what our plan was. Her response was, "Don't ever trust those varmints, they have a terrible reputation." It was too late anyway; the ink had dried.

Regardless of our dismay and disappointment, we had developed the formula for success that could and would be repeated elsewhere. And indeed it was. There are numerous examples worldwide, but one of the most exciting is that of Dr. Armando Lobato from Sao Paulo, Brazil.

He spent two years with us and learned every little trick that we had garnered over the years. The synergy was contagious, and when he left for his home, we had to take inventory of what little was left on the shelves. I have visited him on numerous occasions. He has created the most successful endovascular program in his country, training maybe 75% of the physicians. His annual meeting, CICE, challenges the best in the world. He is just one of the thousands who passed through our program on their own way to an exciting specialty career.

At the instigation of Mr. Donald B. Reid, friend and fellow surgeon, I was inducted into the Royal College of Physicians and Surgeons

Dr. Lobato being presented a special certificate from me.

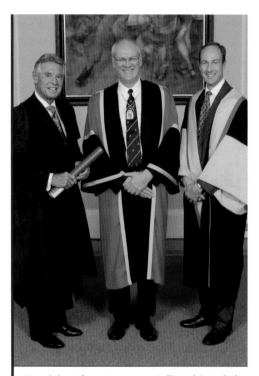

Receiving the Honorary Fellowship of the Royal College of Physicians and Surgeons, wearing Lord Lister's graduation gown from the 1800s. President of the Royal College is Professor Brian Williams (center) beside Donald Reid.

of Glasgow, United Kingdom, on November 17, 2009. King James founded the Royal College of Physicians and Surgeons of Glasgow (RCPSG) in 1599. It is now a multidisciplinary body made up of some 8500 members in the fields of surgery, medicine, and dentistry. The Royal College has a wonderful museum and library. It is still a busy meeting place for physicians and an educational center of excellence and innovation in medicine. It continues to project its sound reputation worldwide. The College is also an historical site, a charity, a place of work, an information provider, and a body that influences governments and public policy. That was indeed a great honor for me.

Honorary Royal Fellowships are given on rare occasions to physicians of outstanding distinction, in one or two small private ceremonies each year. The Royal College council selects the honoree and the President of the Royal College, on behalf of Her Majesty The Queen, presents the Fellowship. As I was to deliver the Lister lecture following my induction, I was given the honor of wearing Lord Lister's original graduation gown, which is over 160 years old. I was told that no one else had put the gown on for over thirty years. Lord Lister was the Regius Professor of Surgery in Glasgow throughout the 1860s; he discovered antiseptic surgery, with the use of carbolic acid.

I delivered the Lister lecture to a large audience of physicians from all over the UK, France, and Ireland. The following evening I was honored by a formal dinner

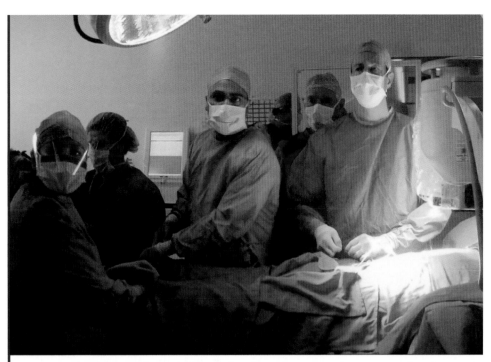

Mr. Donald Reid, President of ISES at the time, demonstrating a case of endovascular repair of a subclavian stenosis. He was proud to show me the skills he had learned in Phoenix, Arizona.

in the Royal College Portrait Gallery. The Surgeon General, Sir Kenneth Calman and Lady Calman, Lord McColl, Lady McColl, Sir Graham and Lady Teasdale, and The Surgical Travellers attended this.

During this same visit, Donald scheduled a few cases at his local hospital.

41

Heart Bike

One of the young artists in our Video Arts Studio, Craig Foster, had the idea of commissioning a custom motorcycle constructed by a famous Arizona designer named Paul Yaffe.

The mission was a "heart" bike—a motorcycle with parts designed to represent the anatomy, instruments, and devices that we used in cardiovascular

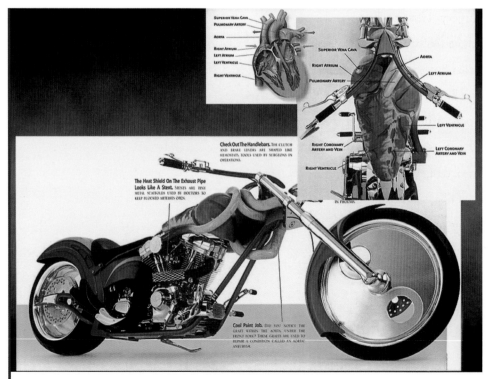

The "Heart Bike" designed by Paul Yaffe. Its major purpose is education and today can be found at the Arizona Science Center.

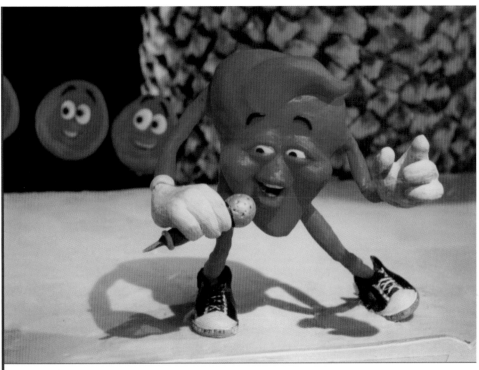

Animated photo of Mr. Heart.

surgery. Ultimately, the bike would be taken to the schools, accompanied by an educator from the Institute, who would talk about the importance of keeping the heart healthy.

For example, the exhaust resembled a stent, the device used to hold the artery open. While pointing to the exhaust pipe, the educator might say, "Smoking causes damage to the lungs and the blood vessels. Don't let that happen to you. Never smoke or you might end up with one of these in your body."

The beautiful bike was a big hit on the school tours. We also had Mr. Heart, a big red heart outfit that one of the staff would wear while performing as the commentator during the visit. The combination was pretty effective in expanding our mission of "Heart Healthy Lessons" for children. Whenever I was with Mr. Heart and the bike, the kids would always ask if I rode it. "Of course!," I'd say, but in reality I only rode it on one short occasion. It was a real piece of art, and I was fearful that it would get scratched up.

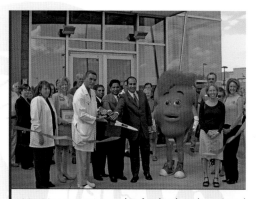

Mr. Heart was popular for both educational and public relations activities as shown here at the opening of the AHI Casa Grande office.

That one exception was during the 2007 International Congress at the Phoenician Resort in Scottsdale. We had the bike on the stage as part of our opening ceremonies. The hotel was not too pleased to have a motorcycle in the ballroom and expressly stated that the engine could not be turned on.

Near the conclusion of the program as I was sitting on the bike, I just could not resist starting the engine. It roared, and I lifted the clutch by mistake. I almost drove off the stage, surrounded by the spontaneous applause of all the colleagues from around the world who thought I had done it on purpose.

What a ride! And there was still more ahead than I could ever imagine, for better or for worse.

42

BT

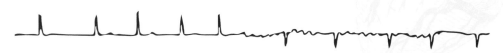

I pushed the overhead button with my right hand and the door opened. Once inside the garage I pushed the second button, again with my right hand. The garage door closed. I reached out with my left hand for the door handle; I could not find it. My hand and arm were groping around the door, and I turned my body toward the left so my right hand could reach the door handle. It was July 17, 2012, Gloria's birthday, and I had just returned home from visiting a clinic in Sun City. While I was tired from my day, I knew something else was wrong. Clumsily, I opened the elevator door and walked in to obtain access to my bedroom. On the ascent I grew nervous and confused. What was happening?

Several years earlier I had an emergency right carotid endarterectomy. *I must be having a recurrence of the carotid disease*, I thought. Upon reaching the bedroom I immediately went to the mirror. I covered my left eye, but there was no vision impairment. The right eye was on the side of the operation, and the right carotid artery also connected to the side of my brain controlling my left arm. I covered my right eye, and I could also see perfectly on that side. It was not a stroke, at least not one caused by carotid artery narrowing. Now I was very anxious. I made a call to one of my staff who was to have a meeting with me explaining, "I'm having a stroke and it's not my carotid." Within less than five minutes a car was there to pick me up.

"Where do you want to go? To the Heart Hospital where Dr. Rodriguez did your carotid endarterectomy?"

"No, to Barrows Neurological Institute. I'm having a stroke."

The last thing I remember was the stroke ER team beginning to work on me; the rest was a nightmare. Seizure activity. A CT scan to rule out an intracranial bleed. The MRI examination, where every cell in my body was shaking uncontrollably. Cold, so very cold. Then…silent peace.

Later when I became fully conscious, I learned they had to sedate me heavily. I recognized my family and could move my arms and legs, but I was still very confused.

Shortly after I was fully awake, a neurologist came into the room and explained my condition. I had a brain tumor (BT) on the right side of the brain, about four inches above my ear. First it would have to be removed, and then they would determine what further therapy would be needed. Not a great birthday present for Gloria; surgery was scheduled for July 19, 2012.

The neurosurgeon Dr. Nakaji must have done a good job removing the brain tumor because, upon awakening, my own neurologic assessment indicated no deficits. Following the surgery, a second physician introduced himself as my neuro-oncologist.

"The tumor is an oligodendroglioma," he explained. "You will need radiation and chemotherapy. We will set up the protocol to start when the incision is healed." Quick. Blunt. Right to the point.

My entire life has been a series of sequels just like that, only about the heart and blood vessels. *At least I'm alive,* I thought. But then a cold hard fact entered my already injured brain. "Your career as a cardiovascular surgeon has just ended."

That was a very devastating moment for me. Was I surprised? No. I had anticipated that. Brain tumors are evil monsters. I showed no emotion. I was just Ted acting like Ted—the pattern of my life.

While on rounds with his residents, Dr. Robert Spetzler stopped by to see me. It was kind of the Chief of Barrow's Neurological Institute (BNI) to make a special visit like that. Before leaving the room he said, "We will take this just one step at a time, Ted." I had already made my mind up to do that very thing. I have learned in my life to accept the worst and construct new options. The frustrating circumstance in this situation was the lack of information. No matter with whom I spoke at BNI, the answer was always the same: it's a cancer. We don't know how it will respond to treatment, and neither do we know the prognosis.

That was just not good enough for me, so I began my own investigation. I read hundreds of pages of information on the subject. I interviewed a world-renowned naturalist in Tucson, Arizona. She was extremely helpful, more so than most of the papers I studied. She was very high on the ketogenic diet and sent me a great deal of information, including recipes. The diet eliminated all sugar; cancer loves sugar.

On my first visit back with the neuro-oncologist at Barrow's after the suggestion regarding the ketogenic diet, I asked what his thoughts were regarding its potential benefits. His response was abrupt. "We have no evidence that there is any benefit from that diet program." It is now three years since that conversation, and my latest MRI shows no tumor.

Recently, a neurologist looking at the MRI said. "It's pristine. Whatever you are doing, keep it up." I mentioned the ketogenic diet. "Oh yes, at our recent tumor board meeting, we initiated a new study describing a special diet for brain tumor patients." Critical point! Patients must be their own advocates in this complex arena of medical care delivery.

The nutritionist also suggested I contact Dr. Mark Rosenberg in Florida. I did, sending him what information I had, and then scheduled a Skype consultation. Now I was beginning to obtain a much better perspective on the cancer culprit. For the first time some of my questions were at least partially answered, the primary one being, "Are there any other treatments I should consider?" He agreed with the chemotherapy, but suggested there were others in the arsenal if needed. I jumped on one of his suggestions.

He said that in the Division of Hematology and Medical Oncology at Weill Cornell Medical Center in New York, Dr. John Boockvar was investigating a vaccine for brain tumors, and I might be a candidate. Within twenty-four hours I was speaking on the phone with Dr. Boockvar at Cornell, and three days later I had an appointment with him. I was determined to pursue the path as fast as possible.

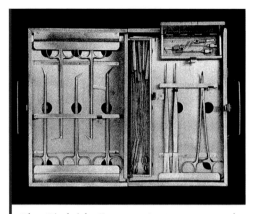

The Diethrich Coronary Instrument set developed by Codman.

As I was standing at the registration desk for my appointment, I saw a stack of medical records with a note on the top that read "Appointments for Dr. Michael Kaplitt." Unbelievable! Michael was a neurosurgeon at Cornell. I had visited him a few years earlier when we were working on a gene project. His father, Marty, was one of my best friends in the early days of heart surgery. He and his colleagues developed the concept of carbon dioxide gas endarterectomy to remove plaque from an artery during a bypass procedure; the technique became common in my operating rooms later on, particularly when the intraoperative angiogram could be used with our new equipment in the hybrid suite, permitting immediate assessment of the procedure. A special retractor with radiopaque blades was needed to permit completely unobstructed angiographic imaging. Codman Instrument Company was helpful in developing the tools required for these innovative procedures, and I prepared a brochure illustrating the operative technique.

What a serendipitous moment! When I met Dr. Boockvar, I asked about Michael, and indeed they were partners in the department of neurosurgery and also shared research space. He told me the FDA vaccine protocol was closed. Results had not been as good as anticipated anyway.

"Is there anything else you can suggest?" I asked. Dr. Boockvar went on to describe a technique under investigation in which a catheter is introduced into the groin artery and threaded up into the neck. It is then inserted directly into the brain to the artery that supplies blood in the area where the brain tumor was just removed.

The Diethrich reverse circumflex scissor was a specialty item, still used today.

The concept was that if there were any remaining or newly developing cancer cells, the chemotherapy drug could be injected through the catheter into the specific site. He did not need to explain this much further. For the past several years, I had been an advocate of delivering agents through catheters and indeed performed procedures where a catheter-based technology was used.

In my case, the area where the tumor had formed was removed months ago, so one key question remained: Would I be a candidate? The decision came like a whirlwind. Marty Kaplitt called his

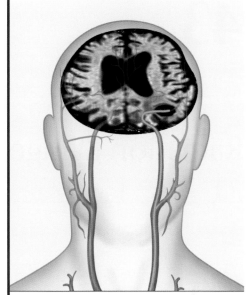

Illustration by Mike Austin showing the catheter placement for the investigative chemotherapy procedure I received while in New York.

son, Michael, who obviously had spoken with Dr. Boockvar, and before I knew it I was on the operating schedule for Tuesday. It was already Friday, the Friday before Thanksgiving. I had to put the brakes on.

Even with everything happening to me, I had to be home for Thanksgiving. It was a big occasion in our family, and at that point they did not know about this latest development. Plus, I doubted the Cornell Hospital's turkey would be up to my standards.

I returned for the operation the week following Thanksgiving. It proceeded without a hitch, and I left the hospital later the same day. Most people travel to New York during the holiday season for Christmas shopping; I went for brain surgery.

Since then, every two months, Dr. Boockvar receives the results of my MRIs performed at BNI and adds an entry in his research file. It is interesting how my life has been altered. I used to think of how I was living from birthday to birthday. Now I think of living from MRI to MRI.

43

Radiation Danger Exposed!

As I was still recuperating from my first brain surgery in 2012, a thought came to me. As you remember, I was very excited about the revolutionary ceiling-mounted angiographic equipment from Germany that we had installed in the operating suite at St. Joe's Hospital in the '70s. It truly was the impetus for the endovascular revolution that followed. A unique feature was the fact that surgeons, not cardiologists or radiologists, were performing the radiographic procedures. We surgeons had been lectured about radiation from the equipment (called scatter) and also how to reduce exposure. Quite honestly, we were not nearly as compelled to wear the radiation protection garments as our colleagues in other disciplines.

They were more aware of the negative effects of radiation.

I learned this the hard way. I had experienced right and left eye cataracts

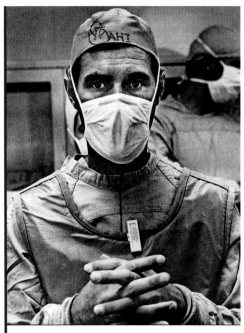

Note the lead apron with the radiation badge. More important, notice the absence of any lead protection around the neck, no lead lined glasses to protect the eyes and no headgear for protection of the brain.

that required operations, the highly calcified plaque in my right carotid artery that required an operation, and now, a right-sided brain tumor. I began to wonder if all of these were consequences of radiation exposure. Was this the common denominator in my personal case? I have documented scientific evidence for cataracts and radiation effects on arteries and, more recently, on brain tumors. It will definitely be an area of my research in the future.

During the Veith meeting in November 2013, I had a conversation with Prof. Peter Fitzgerald, a cardiologist at Stanford University, regarding

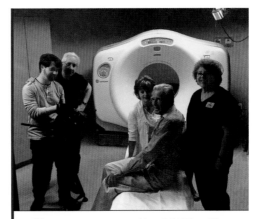

Trillium was contacted by ORSIF to film me as an example of a physician who has been exposed to many years of low dose ionizing radiation scatter in the procedure rooms. From left, Yari and Cary Wolinsky, Penny Hattley who was my secretary for many years and is now the manager of Insight Imaging—Biltmore, where she continues to exhibit her executive skills, Cindy DiPiazza, and me (Dr. John Karis, neuroradiologist read the MRI).

our common interest in the adverse consequences of radiation. I told him of my brain tumor follow-up. He then described to me the Organization for Occupational Radiation Safety in Interventional Fluoroscopy (ORSIF). The organization contacted me, I'm sure as a result of my conversation with Peter. In addition, ORSIF referred a film company called Trillium, a father (Cary) and a son (Yari) partnership, from Norwell, MA, and arrangements were made to produce a documentary film on this particular subject.

The filming for the video segment that ORSIF used to introduce the concept of protection against the chronic low dose radiation exposure was an interesting production in itself. The goal was to produce a five-minute film using me as the model, a living example of the ill effects radiation can have on the human body. The team was in Phoenix for about a week. Their vast film experience was soon obvious and greatly appreciated by all the contributors to the production.

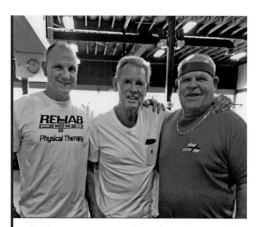

Chad Dunn, me, and Andy Miller; staff at Rehab Plus.

We were predominantly in clinical facilities. The Trillium duet were so professional, their quiet presence was barely noticed. At Biltmore Imaging, Penny Hattley enlisted Dr. John P. Karis, a neurologist, and his technician, Cindy DiPiazza, to provide the scene for MRI imaging and diagnosis of the brain tumor. The absence of the actual brain tumor was made clearly apparent on the screen. Similarly, demonstration of the radiation exposure to the lens of the eye resulting in cataracts and the need for implants was dramatically documented at the Barnett Dulaney Perkins Eye Center in Phoenix, Arizona, where Dr. Perkins himself conducted an examination of my implanted lens for Trillium to film. Filming the OR scene where the radiation scatter is so prevalent was created with the help of Tedd Brandon and Tony Forner of our staff. The all-important reference to the need for rehabilitation secondary to the chronic use of heavy lead protection aprons and long hours in the hybrid operating room was filmed in the Rehab Plus facility operated by Warren Anderson, who you might remember was the trainer of my football team in Chicago and Phoenix.

Once the ORSIF film was released, the genie was out of the bottle. The problems of radiation imaging were suddenly exposed everywhere. Most recently I reviewed a paper from London, UK, that pointed out how the radiation problem, particularly to the head, may become even more prevalent. The completion of the latest endovascular treatment approaches to aortic disease has created radiation exposure times, which can be escalated by angulation of the C-Arm to obtain various views. This may not be widely appreciated but certainly adds an increased risk to the operator. Head protection during these procedures has not been addressed with any intensity. It's unclear at present where this road will lead us, but it may surely mandate a *SLED* exploration in the future.

When I was approached by ORSIF about the potential adverse consequences of radiation, I had completely forgotten my early 1963 study where we were concerned that patients with breast cancer who were receiving chemotherapy and simultaneous radiation treatments might suffer from adverse skin consequences from combined therapy. I developed a protocol to study this issue using a rabbit model. The results of the study were presented at the competition of the regional meeting of the American College of Surgeons. I received the Frederick A. Coller award for this scientific research. This no doubt left some impression on Dr. Coller when many

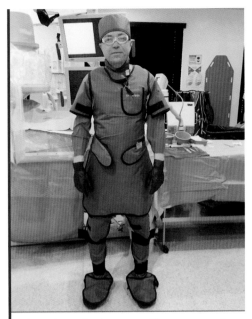

This photo looks more like a scene from *Star Wars* than from a medical angiography laboratory, but clearly he is advocating a religion of total body protection. If the vascular practice fails he is certainly ready for the first charter to the moon!

years later I spoke to him about my Houston application. It also exhibited my early concern that in our therapeutic approach to care, we minimize the potential for harm.

One of my former vascular fellows, (Dr. Mitar Vranic), has created an ambulatory surgical center in the East Valley. This story is about his experience with excessive radiation in a former mentor and is an important testimony to how this problem must be addressed.

During his first vascular fellowship, Dr. Vranic's program director would only wear pelvic and thyroid lead protection during vascular procedures. He subsequently developed an aggressive form of myeloma, non-responsive to treatment, leading to his death. Dr. Vranic decided to hire a radiation expert to measure radiation levels during multiple procedures. The protection program he adopted after this consultation resulted in a dramatic reduction of radiation levels measured by his badges in comparison to previous years.

44

Reflections, Forty Years Past

In 2012, my son Tad planned a "surprise" event at the local resort during the International Congress. He brought together current and past employees, as well as staff and friends from home and abroad. Many stood and told stories about their association with our program and me. It was a moving event, punctuated by Tad presenting me a very special trophy.

He had designed it himself, and in doing so capsulated that same triad I have referred to so many times throughout this book: my music, sports, and work. He described it perfectly with something that portrayed my continued efforts to always create the "team." The name on the trophy read, "The leader of the band." I can never thank him enough for that great evening and the trophy, which sits on the corner of my desk as a daily reminder of my wonderful life's ride and my son's thoughtfulness. My accomplishments, no matter how small they may have been, would not have been possible without my wonderful patients, colleagues, and friends in the worldwide medical community. However, as important as they are, it's apparent to me now that these contributions pale in comparison to the love and support from my family. A splendid example is Tad's gift, Gloria's ever-lasting dedication and love, and Lynne's devotion in the face of negative headlines.

From the earliest days when I would rush off after an ambulance siren to the hospital, leaving Gloria dateless, to the startling recent episode of the brain tumor, she has always been with me, always supported me, even during the worst period of

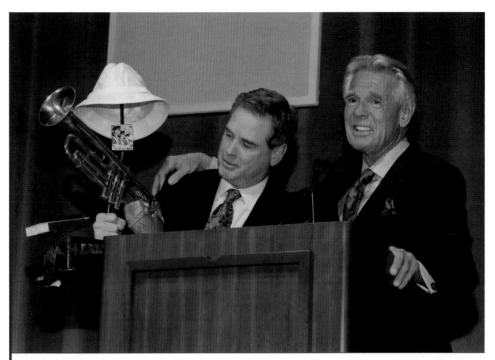

Special trophy presented to me by my son, Tad, at an AHF special tribute event during our annual Congress meeting in 2012. He developed a palpable composite of many of my life's activities.

the Great War with the Medical Mafia. I did not realize how much I appreciated this until recently, when I asked her what material she might have that I could use in this book. A few days later, a large table in my study was filled with files, all carefully labeled and many even with footnotes. Newspaper clippings were perfectly organized in sequence, taking into account activities from high school to the present.

As I read these one by one, for the first time I was struck by how much

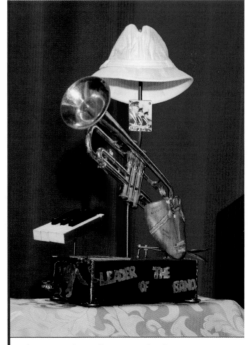

The actual trophy, a work of art.

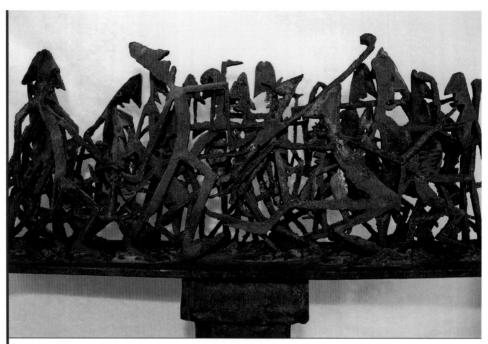

Gloria's gift depicting a typical day in her husband's life.

she must have suffered. Gloria had to see the attacks on her husband in the daily headlines of the local paper, spewed forth from my jealous competitors. She had to face her friends, and it must have been extremely difficult to defend me at her weekly Bridge Club luncheons. Yet, I never heard a single negative word from her. Without her support and encouragement, my career would not have been successful, and I certainly could not have written this book. She was the glue that held the family together and was largely responsible for bringing up Tad and Lynne when I was absent with work.

It was not easy for the kids either. I remember early one morning when Lynne called me at the office after seeing the headlines in the newspaper: "Daddy, I still love you." I am sure Tad had to face abuse from his classmates, some obvious, some subtle.

In going through Gloria's files, I came across a letter from Dr. John Pittman, a thoracic surgical resident while I was at Michigan. We became friends, and he later helped me with the local detractors. The letter was addressed personally to Tad and Lynne:

CARDIOVASCULAR SURGEONS, INC.

THORACIC AND CARDIOVASCULAR SURGERY

HARRY SIDERYS, M.D.
JOHN N. PITTMAN, M.D.
GILBERT T. HEROD, M.D.
HAROLD HALBROOK, M.D.

PROFESSIONAL OFFICES
1815 N. CAPITOL AVENUE
INDIANAPOLIS, INDIANA 46202

BUSINESS OFFICE
1815 N. CAPITOL AVENUE
INDIANAPOLIS, INDIANA 46202

PHONE 317-923-1787

DONALD P. WATTS
Manager

March 30, 1976

Lynne and Tad Diethrich
4819 East Humming Bird Lane
Scotsdale, Arizona 85253

Dear Lynne and Tad,

As I am sitting at my home study looking out toward the barn on this stormy morning, I can't help but see a giant oak tree between our house and barn. During this storm, when the wind is shaking the foundation and limbs of this giant old oak tree, one can't help but reflect over the similarities between man and tree. The roots of the tree represent our religious, moral and educational beliefs which constitute our higher brain powers. The trunk of the tree represents our bodies. Each tiny limb of the tree is reaching out into space. The buds are now appearing and the real life process of the tree is about to explode into a fantastic array of leaves, and all of this is guided by the brainy root system. Our limbs are our eyes, ears, fingers and mouth which are exposed to the weather. The weather in Phoenix has been quite stormy. But you know, there is always clean, fresh, fragrant air and calm that follows a storm. The storm is passing from Phoenix, and you will soon note clean air.

As a father of five children, I am concerned as are your parents about the atmosphere in which our children are raised. You two have been exposed to a large number of newspaper articles which have not flattered your father. In the clean air that follows the storm, this will change.

I have spent seven days of my life listening to a lot of testimony against your Dad. Let me assure you that none of the surgeons in the world would enjoy the experience that your Dad has been subjected to. The Monday morning quarterbacks are everywhere. Indiana might lose to U.C.L.A. today. If so, many people will say they lost because Bobby Knight didn't do something right.

A heart surgeon has an exposure similar to a coach. If something goes wrong he is responsible. The big difference is that a coach is the director of some of the most superb specimens of mankind that exist. A heart surgeon is dealing with people whose bodies are frequently weak and frail as a result of their long standing illness. It is difficult to have an undefeated season with that kind of a team of players. Those players, though weak, have more courage than Kent Bentson. They are playing a gambling game with their lives at stake. If they win, their life is better. If they lose, they might be dead. No athlete faces those odds.

One of the accusations against your Dad was that he was coaching (operating) too many bad players (patients). Any heart surgeon who is worth his salt would have taken this same coaching job.

In my opinion, your Dad is guilty of being an excellent surgeon with the endurance and drive of three men. He is guilty of loving his wife and two children. You are lucky to have him for a father. I am fortunate to have him for a friend.

Sincerely,

JOHN N. PITTMAN, M. D.

Dr. Pittman died on Christmas Day 2014. His death was a great sadness to my family.

At this time, I do not recall if I originally saw the letter. However, I am sure Gloria did and discussed it with the children. Reading it now reinforces my earlier comment regarding true friends: the finger count.

I have been fortunate to receive many awards and honors during my career. In looking over Gloria's clippings, I ran across this address I gave on June 2, 1974, to the 100th graduating class of my alma mater high school in Hillsdale.

The address, titled "The Challenge of Graduation," is appropriate today, even though it's forty years later. It concerns me that the lessons and admonitions I alluded to in the address have fallen on deaf ears in many instances:

THE CHALLENGE OF GRADUATION

It is a great pleasure for me to return to Hillsdale, my home for eighteen years and to participate in this centennial graduation from my own high school. It seems impossible that two decades have passed since I have walked the halls of what now is the old high school, played on the athletic fields and sang our own song, "The Maize and Blue." Time has marched on these past twenty years and now you have new facilities, expanded programs and most certainly, progressive and innovative educational ambitions. I am sure, however, that there remains the same tradition of excellence in education, with a strong commitment to the words which were inscribed over the entrance of my former school:

"Enter to learn—Go forth to serve."

You, the members of the graduating class, have had the opportunity of four years of secondary education leading up to this day—the day of your commencement. You can be proud of your achievements—the accomplishments you have made academically, in athletics, in music, and other extracurricular activities. And we the alumni, the faculty, and your parents and friends are justly proud of you and give you our congratulations on your record of accomplishments.

But may I hasten, before you become disillusioned with too much praise, that today represents not the end, not the finale of your life's record of achievements, but the beginning. Today is the commencement of an entirely new life for each of you.

This new life will commence in a world drastically changed from the one my graduating class faced twenty years ago. The world which once was expansive, separated geographically by oceans and lacking rapid communication and transportation, has now been compacted to an unbelievably tiny sphere. Europe, the Far and Middle East, all two decades ago seemed as far away as the moon. Yet today, they are within reach in a few short hours. The significance of this global shrinkage upon your future cannot be minimized because now, more than ever before, America and its people will be influenced and affected by decisions and actions from our friends and, unfortunately, in many cases, those not so friendly to us, from around the world.

You must be prepared to not only face the challenges before you in our own country, but also those presented by other nations. I have just returned two weeks ago from a trip to the Middle East countries of Saudi Arabia and Jordan and I can assure you that I have real concern for the future of our land. In contrast to those young developing countries, we have lived through years of bountiful plenty. You, the members of this graduating class of 1974 are the products of this generation and I believe it would be a correct assessment to state that very few, if any of you, have ever really been challenged to your capabilities. Life has been comfortable for you. Your education, your food, your clothing, your pleasures, have been attended to. There have never been bombs and destruction, or fleeing for your lives. You have never been subjected to the ravages of disease and poverty that I observed abroad.

Indeed, for many of you, major decisions may have been selection of the proper TV channel for your evening amusement and in some cases, even that was probably accomplished by a remote control "space command" push button device.

If you believe these observations to be somewhat harsh and, perhaps unexpected on this your special day, let me assure you that this is not a condemnation of this graduating class, but a concern for our future as a people and a country. Great and powerful countries and civilizations have fallen before—in fact, on that same Middle East trip I saw evidences of what was once the Great Roman Empire and I could not help but think perhaps its people, too, became the object of "easy living."

While it would appear on the surface that you begin your journey into this new life with many advantages, it is possible that your development to this point in fact may represent, in some instances, an increased burden for you, not as a result of any of your own doing, but rather our society's own laissez-faire attitudes. You will, in my opinion, be called upon to rise to greater heights than any graduating class before you because the challenges of this and subsequent decades will be greater than ever before experienced.

For example, you have witnessed over the past twenty-four months an incredible destruction in the credibility of our American leadership. It is not my intention to judge the merits of our governmental representatives' actions, first because it would be a futile exercise in suppositions, and secondly, it would have to be based on other than first-hand documented evidence. But it is vital that you as new graduates about to embark on the most important adventure of your lives, realize fully the impact which these most unfortunate events will have on your future. Not only has the reputation of Washington been tarnished, but also the esteemed position of the United States of America as a leader in the arena of world affairs has suffered.

As impossible as it may seem to you today, it is entirely possible that during your lifetime you will witness a situation where our country either is *sharing* a world leadership role or perhaps even more desperately, finds itself in a secondary position.

Your future will be played on a stage with this backdrop of national and international crises in a period of political, social and economic fluctuation.

A few moments ago, I spoke about your academic preparation to this point and the fact that few if any of you have been inspired to reach your potential. As you begin a new role in life, you will find it increasingly important to set your goals and aspirations at the highest levels—in spite of the numerous obstacles, which will face you. The greatest tragedy of our times and one, which must be corrected and avoided at all costs if your personal future and the future of your country are to flourish, is the strong tendency toward mediocrity which permeates our society.

As I reflect on my own career since graduation from this high school, I recall many times when there was an opportunity or tendency for mediocre rather than excellent performance. So frequently in our daily lives the mediocre course of action seems most expedient-less troublesome and in general "an easier way."

Mediocrity begets mediocrity, and one cannot expect anything better, or more challenging—if one's level of performance and ambitions are only average.

Many of the problems which I alluded to, and to which you will have to address yourselves to in the future, have been created out of an environment in which we have not set our goals high enough—in which we have sold short our true potential. It would be a great tragedy if any member of this graduating class failed to achieve his total potential and capability.

In my profession, my staff and I at the Heart Institute are faced each day with life and death issues.

A man's heart that is about to be rendered useless by a heart attack.

A young child born with a cardiac abnormality that prevents normal growth and development.

A youthful mother suffering from a defective heart valve—unable to care for her growing children.

I am sure each of you can realize that in the correction and care of these health problems, there is no place for mediocre performance—yet medicine is but one example of the many jobs and professions available to you where a standard of quality is so important to the end product. Unless you are constantly on the alert however, mediocrity will creep into even your thinking.

I charge you to meet the challenges before you by setting your standards high. Do not accept less than that which is perfect and let excellence rather than mediocrity be your measurement of success. When faced with difficult and frustrating situations, shun away from taking the path of least resistance. Rather, accept adversity for what it is yet another opportunity to develop, mature, and reach your total potential.

Graduates of the Class of 1974, the centennial class of Hillsdale High School, we, your family and friends, wish you success as you commence on your new journey. The greatness of your achievements in life will be limited only by your personal commitment and dedication. Congratulations and best wishes as you "go forth to serve."

The discovery of this graduation address in Gloria's files may be the ultimate serendipitous event related to this book project. It epitomizes my life story, without portraying a narrative of events; however, I do not want to minimize those in any way. In reality it's about my philosophy of life, which has always been my guiding compass.

My appointment as a member of the National Advisory Board for the Cardiovascular Center of the University of Michigan afforded me a unique opportunity to interact with faculty and become acquainted with research and educational activities at my alma mater. I visited the north campus where the research laboratories of Professor Ramon Berguer and Tom Wakefield were being established. This represented a real transformation from the early days of the dog lab experiences at St. Joe's down the street to the modern era of laboratory research at a major university. Throughout my career, and particularly my experience at Baylor College of Medicine, my research reflected a common theme of exploring instrumentation development for use in treating disease in the cardiovascular system. Maybe a special gene surfaced early in my life that continues its expression to this day.

Two years ago I was contacted by some members of the Michigan faculty with the suggestion of creating an endowment for a new Professorship in the Department of Biomedical Engineering and Section of Vascular Surgery, Department of Surgery at the University of Michigan. I did not jump at the idea because memoirs and legacies have always been for me like engravings on the tombstone, and I'm not yet ready for that resting place. There was, however, a bump in the road between creating the concept and actual execution.

Universities are comprised of various schools; nursing, law, public health, engineering and so forth. Most often these schools function like silos with a dean or leader and various department heads who are responsible for the section under their authority. An example would be the head of the department of surgery overseeing the sections of neurosurgery, thoracic surgery, and so forth. This traditional structure has been in existence for a long time, but recently it appears to be at least somewhat dysfunctional.

The endovascular movement has demanded the establishment of more flexibility and ultimately closer cooperation between these section heads and certainly the department heads. As an example, complex endovascular procedures may require a working cooperation between vascular and cardiac surgeons, cardiologists,

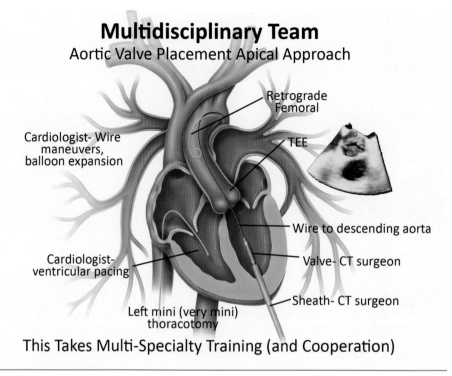

Multidisciplinary Team
Aortic Valve Placement Apical Approach

Retrograde Femoral

Cardiologist- Wire maneuvers, balloon expansion

TEE

Wire to descending aorta

Cardiologist- ventricular pacing

Valve- CT surgeon

Sheath- CT surgeon

Left mini (very mini) thoracotomy

This Takes Multi-Specialty Training (and Cooperation)

This drawing illustrates in detail the multi-specialists who are involved in complex endovascular procedures.

and radiologists applying their unique skills and knowledge for a successful procedure. I have recognized this phenomenon for many years and historically that was why I led the ISES organization to engage all of these specialties in response to the projected vision for the endovascular evolution.

Throughout this time I have been intrigued by the concept of amalgamation. A unification of physicians clearly had to occur. This would also include the technicians and parallel staff. Ideally the process of amalgamation of two disciplines would be employed to create useful and safe expansion of technologies as they were rolled out. My vision was that perhaps all of this could be hastened through a formal structure at Michigan.

Tom Wakefield, MD, current Professor and Section Head of Vascular Surgery and one of the Directors of the Cardiovascular Center; Jim Stanley, MD (remember him from the St. Joe's lab days?), Professor of Vascular Surgery and previous Section

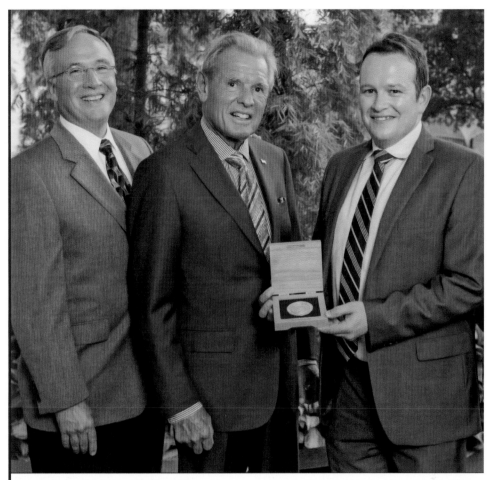

James Woolliscroft, Dean of the University of Michigan Medical School, me, and Alberto Figueroa, the newly appointed Professor of Biomedical Engineering and Vascular Surgery.

Head and former Director of the Cardiovascular Center; Michael Mulholland, MD, Head of the Department of Surgery and Professor Ramon Berguer, among many others, were helpful and successful in establishing the Professorship and selecting its first recipient. James Woolliscroft, MD, Dean of the Medical School, was an enthusiastic supporter throughout the process.

On May 18, 2015, Dr. C. Alberto Figueroa was inaugurated as the first recipient of the Edward B. Diethrich Research Professorship in Biomedical Engineering and Vascular Surgery. He is an outstanding young scientist with a clear vision that the future melding of science and medical practice in the endovascular field must

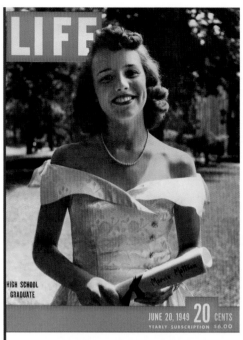

Marsha Mattson on the cover of *LIFE*.

occur. This professorship was a synthesis of the amalgamation concept. I believe this appointment is unique and could be the first of its kind in the United States.

It was a warm feeling that day to know that many of the projects I had worked on and many more that were only in my mind might someday come to fruition under a Professorship I had helped to create.

In late February of 2015, my long-time friend Phil Kneen emailed that he and his wife would be traveling through Phoenix in March and would like to stop by for a visit. I was delighted. Phil and I had been friends beginning in grade school until he went east to Cornell and I went to Ann Arbor. We were partners in the acappella trio of the choir, played football and basketball, and shared the excitement of the band and orchestra. When I talked to him on the phone prior to his visit, I suggested that he bring along any photos, papers, or memorabilia of our early days together that would be good for the *SLED* production. Most important, when I told him about the *LIFE* magazine article regarding the Institute and the trouble it had created for me, he recalled the story when *LIFE* magazine came to Hillsdale and did an article on a typical Midwestern town in the United States. Phil brought a copy of the publication for me. It was unbelievable because I had truly forgotten all about it.

I was definitely not a key figure in the Hillsdale story, but there was an article on the front cover featuring Marsha Mattson.

She was the beautiful daughter of Dr. Frazier Mattson, who was the surgeon I observed many years before when my mother was scrubbing in the OR for him.

As I mention earlier, Dr. Mattson communicated with me regarding the televised live heart operation.

I have always met challenges before me by setting the highest standards possible. Accepting less than perfection and excellence was not in the plan. Likewise, accepting mediocrity as a solution to a difficult problem was not tolerable.

Yes, I set my personal goals and ambitions at the highest level, just as I had challenged the graduating students. What I failed to properly convey to them were the consequences you have read about in my book: some good and some potentially lethal.

Throughout my life's journey I have found it vital to explore every road, and not every one was an expressway. In fact, there are some bumps, many curves, and treacherous turns to be negotiated. From time to time, the reality was to face a wreck that either I or someone else had created. Regardless, every trail must be explored because one never knows what the exploration of another path may offer, even those with railroad crossings.

45

Another Railroad Track

The ride is over, the last bump was not conquered; it was just too tough! I was a little slow in recognizing a problem with Tympani. On our daily morning and evening walks she was always ten yards or so in front of me. Her head held high, sniffing the bushes and her tail wagging in sync with the pace. Over a period of three to four weeks, I noticed she was lagging behind, I thought looking for a rabbit under the bushes. However, she suddenly did not care about walking with me and her appetite disappeared. It was time for a vet checkup with Dr. Bracken. He called quickly and informed me that Tympani was anemic and needed a bone marrow study by Dr. Hoffman a specialist. This was accomplished in a couple of days and accompanied by a two-pint blood transfusion. The bone marrow report was not encouraging. Tympani had immune mediated hemolytic anemia and needed steroid treatment. That program was initiated, but with only mildly positive results. She was weak and without an appetite even for the treat that I provided with meals, which of course was forbidden.

It was very early Thursday morning, and I was preparing to leave for Houston to present a keynote lecture for Dr. Coselli's Current Trends meeting. Tympani was lying very quietly on the floor next to my bed. I lay down next to her, head to head, which was not unusual. Frequently, I had whispered conversations with her, particularly on travel days, like, "I am going to be gone for a few days but you will be fine." This whispered conversation was difficult. Her eyes did not have the usual sparkle. I could see her respirations were somewhat labored. I told her she was going to be just okay. Neither of us believed that at all. She looked at me and turned her head to the floor. I knew it was time for our final conversation, "Tympani, what name do you suggest for the new puppy?" From somewhere came the response, "Keep it in the rhythm section!" That was our last conversation. The new puppy will be named Cymbals, consistent with Tympani's wishes and the musical connotations in the *SLED* story.

Good sledding, my friends!

Hi, I'm Cymbals, guide for your next ride! Hang on tightly; it's going to be wonderful!

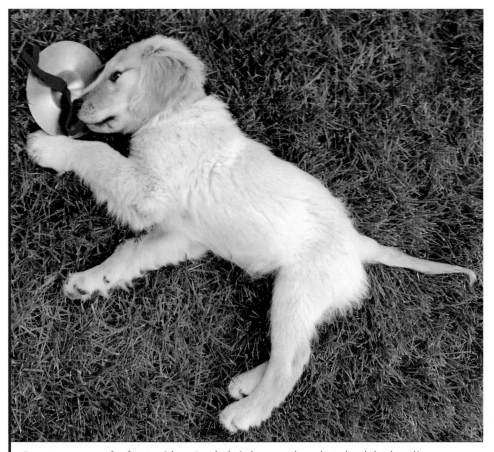

Our new mascot for future rides, Cymbals is here and ready to lead the band!

46

What If?

Seemingly, it never ends… speaking of course, of serendipity. I was in the neurosurgeon's office, discussing with Dr. Nakaji my latest MRI scan. It had been four months since the prior scan when no residual tumor was found. However, on the current scan, an area of suspicious scar tissue was observed. He called me over to the viewing screen where the scan performed the day before was projected.

"We have some questions about this area, which before was considered scar tissue. There are findings that could relate to post-treatment change versus tumor recurrence. Even though you've had no symptoms and your neurologic exam is negative, it is my recommendation we remove that area for histologic examination. This will help us determine if any other therapy might be required."

It seemed perfectly logical to me, and I asked him to set up the procedure at his earliest convenience.

As he was leaving the room, he said, "Oh Ted, just one other thing. We have a new research protocol using fluorescein, which we inject at the time of the operation. This dye differentiates the scar tissue from potential tumor tissue. The tumor lights up in an orange-yellow color. This is a new technique, and we don't have a lot of experience with it, but in a few cases it has been helpful. It is low risk. Would you be interested?"

"Absolutely, sign me up!"

"Good, I'll send the research nurse in to sign the forms, see you soon."

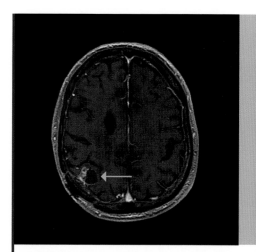 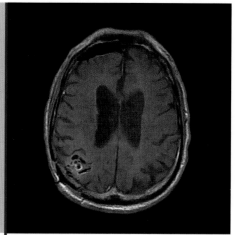

MRI depicting suspicious area of possible recurrent tumor (8/19/15).

MRI picture after removal of suspicious area (8/20/15).

The procedure was scheduled for the next afternoon. The research nurse did not come and see me before I left the hospital. There was a later phone message that she had called about the protocol, but I did not talk with her.

In the morning I had a call informing me that the procedure had been moved up two hours on the schedule, so I quickly prepared to go to the hospital and checked into the preoperative area. I signed more consents, undressed, and stretched out on the bed where an IV was started. OR nurses and the anesthesiologist came in for introductions and last minute questions. Yes, even the orderly to wheel me into the operating room came in to say hello. This reminded me of my early days at the Hillsdale Hospital.

I was ready to go when suddenly a nurse introduced herself as the research RN in charge of the fluorescein study. She opened her folder and pulled out the study consent form. The wheels on the stretcher were already rolling. I reached out for the pen and made a scrambled signature as I was waving to the nurses with the other hand. I was flying down the corridor to the OR.

The next afternoon, Dr. Nakaji stopped by to check me before I was to be discharged from the hospital. He showed me the MRI that had been taken at 4 a.m. after the procedure. (Yes, really in the middle of the night. I guess they don't believe postop neuro patients need sleep.) He pointed to the area of the previous scar tissue that had been in question. It was gone!

"I have to tell you Ted, the fluorescein made a real contribution in this case. We were not sure what was scar tissue and what could be new tumor. When we injected the dye, the area in question turned color, suggesting tumor. We resected it, sent it to pathology, and indeed it contained tumor cells. We would never have been able to have that precise differentiation without the tissue stain."

Yes, serendipity in action once again.

What if the research nurse had not appeared and I had not signed the consent? What if the doctor at the last minute had not discussed the fluorescein with me? What if? What if? Yes, it will never end.

Thank You

How did I drive this sled? It's been multiple years since I used the antiquated typewriter. I am essentially part of the computer illiterate generation. So I resorted to ballpoint pen scratched on lined 8½ x 11 pads of paper. These mostly unreadable scribblings were then passed on to my transcribers and then the editors. I needed a quiet place to review their work and I could not have found a better place than the Institute's close friends at Avanti's restaurant. For many years, Benito Mellino and Angiolo Livi brought lunch to the staff at the Institute. These luncheon specials were expertly coordinated by Theresa Capriotti, RN, our clinic director. I even asked Angiolo and Mario for their comments on some of my stories since they were familiar with the Institute's endeavors.

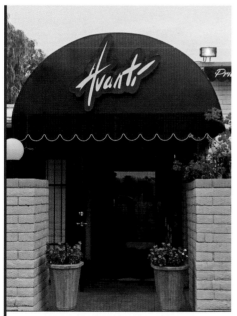

Avanti's restaurant, home of the very best lasagna in the world, better than Italy.

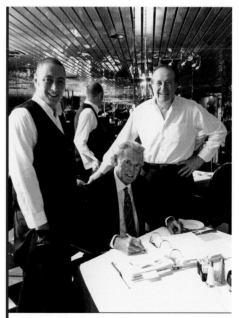

Mario Mellino and Angiolo Livi giving me advice on one of the book chapters.

Index